LAUGHING THROUGH THE TEARS

OF

BREAST CANCER

—My Personal Metamorphosis

Carla Chesser RN

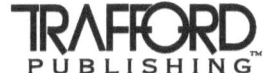

Note for Librarians: A cataloguing record for this book is available from Library and Archives Canada at www.collectionscanada.ca/amicus/index-e.html

ISBN 1-4120-6836-3

Printed on paper with minimum 30% recycled fibre. Trafford's print shop runs on "green energy" from solar, wind and other environmentally-friendly power sources.

TRAFFORD
PUBLISHING™

Offices in Canada, USA, Ireland and UK

This book was published *on-demand* in cooperation with Trafford Publishing. On-demand publishing is a unique process and service of making a book available for retail sale to the public taking advantage of on-demand manufacturing and Internet marketing. On-demand publishing includes promotions, retail sales, manufacturing, order fulfilment, accounting and collecting royalties on behalf of the author.

Book sales for North America and international:

Trafford Publishing, 6E–2333 Government St.,

Victoria, BC V8T 4P4 CANADA

phone 250 383 6864 (toll-free 1 888 232 4444)

fax 250 383 6804; email to orders@trafford.com

Book sales in Europe:

Trafford Publishing (UK) Limited, 9 Park End Street, 2nd Floor

Oxford, UK OX1 1HH UNITED KINGDOM

phone 44 (0)1865 722 113 (local rate 0845 230 9601)

facsimile 44 (0)1865 722 868; info.uk@trafford.com

Order online at:

trafford.com/05-1747

10 9 8 7 6 5 4 3 2

About the Cover

2005© Photograph by Kerry Kelly.
The Tiger Swallowtail butterfly (*Papilio glaucas*) known as a strong flier is distinctive with yellow and black striped markings on its wings and body. It undergoes a complete metamorphosis through four different life stages: egg, caterpillar (larva), pupa (chrysalis), adult butterfly.

This Tiger Swallowtail butterfly has a "nick" in the right wing; however the wound does not detract at all from its beauty.

The photo is symbolic of all women who have undergone their own mutations following surgery from breast cancer...and the metamorphosis that results from this life-altering process.

Acknowledgments

First, I want to acknowledge the Divine Source from Whom all blessings come; giving us what we need—to become who we really are. I am thankful for His continuous blessings during this experience, which I recognized as 'Divine Interventions'. Through these interventions, I believe that I was guided to the make the right decisions and was inspired to accept and overcome this challenge.

Second, I want to acknowledge my daughter Kelly, who before she was even conceived, I knew (in a dream) would be the love of my life. I am grateful that she never treated me any differently during my diagnosis and treatment, though deep down I know she feared for my life.

Third, I appreciate and acknowledge all of the people who have touched my life and shared with me their spiritual gifts and talents; and who offered their love and unconditional emotional, spiritual and physical comfort and support while walking with me on this journey. In addition to my parents, Sara and Ted Baldwin, those members of my family and friends include: Bill, Mercedes and Erin Baldwin; Sandy Bianco; Ann and Kristin Delo; Janis Baldwin; Debi, Terry, Ryan and Megan Hubbard; Trish and Richard Harris; Melinda and Bryan Dorman; Marge, Ed and Justin Brennan; Diana Moore; Nadine and Jessica Lutz; Sue Halloran; Jo and Craig Manion; Kay Taylor; Olga Rasmussen; Sharon Fox; Linda Stone and Alan Beder; Barb Leon; Wendy Wilson; Pat Salmon; Sandy DiBona; Judy Bullock; Jacqueline Flourney; Michelle Lopez; Polette Gardner; Helen Ciallella; Brett Walker; Maureen and Dave Pavlik; Priscilla Ducey; Gay Castor-Fischer; Pat Davis; Jennie Campbell; Patty Jackson; Lynn Dollar; Beth Cochran; Sandy Donnan; Gordon Shuey, Paddy Faucher, Teri O'Shaughnessy, Amy Mecca and Nathan Anspach.

Fourth, I want to recognize the doctors, nurses and other healthcare staff who have dedicated their lives to the care and service of others. I am especially grateful to those who express their compassion and love through their work on a daily basis including Dr. Debra Dube, Dr. Sarah Willard and her nurse Susie; Dr. David Molthrop and Dr. Scott Rotatori and his nurses, Norma and Anne.

Also, I will never forget my very favorite front desk gals at 'The Chemo Place', Kathy Lee and Sally Boomer.

And last but not least, the many people whose names I will never know—those who have prayed for me and wished me well; who smiled at me in the hallways of the hospital, shared words in an elevator and in the lines of a grocery store, providing me the lift that I needed at that particular moment in time. To me, these are my angels on earth.

Dedication

Thank you St. Jude, for the promise of hope
you hold out to all who believe;
please inspire me to give this gift of hope to others as
it has been given to me.

Disclaimer

Medically-related information in this book is the result of careful research that was done while dealing with the diagnosis of breast cancer and its treatment. The information contained within is provided as background only for relating my own personal experience. Decisions that I made throughout this experience may not relate to you or your loved ones' experience with cancer. You should always consult with your own physicians about information that you receive (from any source) and, along with their professional advice, make the best decisions for yourself.

I wish you the very best possible outcome as you begin this journey...as so many before you have done.

—Carla Chesser RN

Table of Contents

Prologue

"No problem can stand the assault of sustained thinking."

—Voltaire

As I sit down to write this book, I think of the thousands of people who this year will hear the words I heard last year: "It's cancer".

It is hard to fathom that every 30 seconds a woman is diagnosed with breast cancer and more than 239,000 women and 2100 men will be diagnosed with breast cancer before the clock strikes midnight on New Year's Eve (American Cancer Society). All of these people will be faced with making decisions about a diagnosis that they didn't ask for, didn't want and—in most cases—certainly didn't expect.

Each will go through the grieving process—starting with SHOCK and hopefully, ending with some type of ACCEPTANCE, or a reasonable facsimile thereof. But one thing is certain...each of their lives and the lives of those around them will be changed forever.

This is a story of change; a "metamorphosis"; a personal story of how the experience of cancer has resulted in my evolving into a being that I never would have become...without the "gift" of cancer. For the rest of my life, this gift will affect me, my family, my friends and everyone else with whom I come in contact.

Shortly after I was diagnosed, I read that God often tries to get our attention by tapping us on the shoulder...if we don't pay attention He will then shake us a little...and, if we still don't respond, He will KICK US IN THE BUTT! For me, cancer was a kick in the butt that *really* got my attention...and with this experience, I have gained so much more than I ever expected.

Cancer has truly enriched my life by opening my eyes to opportunities that I may have been missing. Having cancer has:

—awakened my JOY for living

—enhanced and reinforced my FAITH

—opened my heart to the deep and abiding LOVE for friends and family

—experienced what it's like to ACCEPT and RECEIVE

—tested my sense of HUMOR

Following chemotherapy, I sometimes complained about feeling horrible, wondering if I would ever get 'back to normal'. Hearing this, my boss would say: "Don't worry, when you finish this process, you will get back to normal...but you won't be the same person." He was right. After experiencing cancer, not only am I not the person I was before, but I don't *want* to be that person. Coping with cancer has challenged me to learn who I really am, to change things that no longer work for me and to grow into the person I was intended to be.

The learning began when I first heard the words "You have cancer". Prior to the day I was diagnosed, I never thought about what my reaction to those words might be—because, as you know, "Cancer always happens to someone else".

At that moment, I believe I went into "auto-pilot"—meaning that I reacted to cancer as I have to all the other challenges that I have faced in my life. It was a *subconscious* reaction. And, yes, sometimes a subconscious reaction can be good...but I realized that a reaction is not the same as a decision. A *conscious decision* requires thoughtful awareness and facing a situation head-on. As I thought more about those words "You have cancer", I realized that in order to face my cancer, I had to make a *conscious* choice in answering the question: "*How* am I going to *react* to this diagnosis...and everything that goes with it?"

Do I want to:

1. Lay down and be depressed during the entire process?
—OR—

2. Continue to live my life with vigor and humor and ATITUDE!

I am not saying that I fooled myself into thinking that I would never feel sorry for myself or even get into some sort of funk, but I knew that I didn't want to *wallow* in those feelings. I knew that it would not be good for me, my family or friends—and I knew it would not be good for my body and its natural mechanisms for fighting illness. So, in reading this book, you will see that I made a conscious decision to fight this cancer, knowing I had to do it with a conscious desire to be vital and healthy and strong...and to approach it with some laughter...which, by the way, is good for the immune system.

This book is written with the intention of helping others to feel less frightened about this diagnosis, to acknowledge the *blessings* that come with having this diagnosis, to find things that are *positive* about this diagnosis, to *be open* to learning and teaching and sharing this illness with others, and to *laugh* about situations surrounding the treatment of this diagnosis that are just plain FUNNY. (*Yes, believe me...there are plenty of things to laugh about.*)

Throughout this experience, I have truly recognized the blessings that so many cancer survivors talk about...those that come hand-in-hand with the devastating diagnosis, the difficult decisions, the debilitating treatments, the decisions, the offers of help, the decisions, the prayers, the decisions, the support and the love. (...oh yeah, did I mention the decisions???)

Although I didn't realize it at the time, the idea for this book was conceived during the first few days of my diagnosis. I would get a dozen phone calls each night, from family and friends wanting to know "what was going on, what have I heard, what I was going to do." Before I got off the phone with one person, my phone would beep with another call. After several nights of missing meals and being exhausted from repeating my self over and over again, I told everyone that although I truly appreciated their concern I would get in touch with them *whenever anything of significance happened*...and I would send it via a group email.

And so, the documentation of my experiences began. I put together an email group, naming them: "My Prayer Group". This group included about 35 people with whom I wanted to share this journey. Thirty-five people that I could count on to provide the love, encouragement, support and prayers that I knew I would need in the coming months.

The subject line of the emails was always "Metamorphosis", knowing that this ongoing documentation would not only describe changes that affected me, but also those to whom I wrote.

Indeed, "My Prayer Group" and I have been changed by this experience. If you ask any one of them, they will say that each email—allowing them to see the highlights of this experience from my perspective—was truly a special gift that they all cherish.

Within these pages, I am about to share with you the same things that I shared with family and friends—MY experiences. I am including emails that I sent out over the year-long period of treatment and recovery with many of the responses from my wonderful Prayer Group. Along with that I have included some of my inner thoughts and in-depth comments, in order that you might benefit from a more personal side of cancer. I am also providing information that I personally found to be interesting and helpful as I tried to figure out how to deal with breast cancer and its treatment.

Throughout this book, I am offering a positive and fearless approach to what could otherwise be a devastating experience.

My understanding is that no two people will have the exact same experience when they go through the diagnosis and treatment of breast cancer...and certainly, many will be diagnosed at different stages. But, there are some experiences that we will have in common and hopefully, you can relate to those.

By the way, as you will find out through your own journey, you may have less control during this experience than you would like. However, one thing you can control is your attitude towards it...and if you take it one day at a time, you can continue to laugh through your tears.

1. Finding the "Lump"

God says: "I will direct your steps" —Proverbs 3:5-6

I am a pediatric nurse with a degree in psychology. Not wanting to share my age (the prerogative of every woman), I am younger than many of you and older than some. But, as those of us who have experienced cancer know—it doesn't really matter your age. Cancer imposes itself on the young and the old, the strong and the weak, the healthy and the sick.

Since entering my thirties, I have considered myself to be a strong and fiercely independent woman who is extremely healthy. I exercise in the gym at least three times a week and I maintain a healthy diet. I get regular check-ups and have had a mammogram every year for the past 15 years. My primary care physician would often comment during my annual exam about how "boring" I was, because my blood work was normal, my tests were negative and I wasn't taking any medications other than a multi-vitamin. So, you can imagine my surprise when I was diagnosed with "the big C". Other than fibrocystic (lumpy) breasts, I have virtually none of the risk factors associated with breast cancer. I am not obese, have an active lifestyle and have no family history of breast cancer. But during this experience I learned that approximately *70% of women with breast cancer have no family history, nor any other risk factor.*

Years ago I gave up caffeine (one of the suspected causes of fibrocystic breasts) and routinely checked my breasts for lumps. But it is often difficult to find a 'suspicious' lump when you are cursed with fibrocystic breasts. Therefore, religiously, I had my annual mammograms and said my prayers when the radiologist ordered an additional diagnostic ultrasound for "a closer check".

My story begins in January 2003 during an annual exam, when my primary care doctor—who once again commented on my "extremely lumpy breasts"—thought she felt "something unusual along the milk duct at about 9 o'clock" on my right breast. She ordered a diagnostic ultrasound which turned out to be negative. I was a happy camper when I heard the results and thought nothing more about it.

However, only nine months later, I noticed a "pea-sized" lump located at about 10 o'clock on my right breast under the skin—

so close to the skin that if I pulled my skin tight, I could see the tiny little cyst.

Being a nurse I knew the drill and wasn't going to wait until *after* I saw my doctor to begin what could have taken a month or more to get things scheduled. I called to make an appointment with Dr. Dube, my primary care doctor, and then immediately called to schedule an appointment for a diagnostic ultrasound. I had a little difficulty getting the mammogram and ultrasound scheduled because of the apparent shortage of radiologists in the area.

The conversation with the scheduler went like this…

"Well, we could get you in on January 26th".

"Uhh-h—this is October—I am NOT waiting 3 months—I have a cyst and I want it checked out as soon as possible!!!"

I was trying not to scream at her.

"Do you have a prescription from the doctor?" the scheduler asked.

"No", I replied, "But, by the time I get there, I will have one." *Sheesh, give me a break!!!*

I got off the phone with her and then called to schedule an appointment with a surgeon; satisfied that all three appointments were scheduled within the same week.

C-O-N-T-R-O-L…it has always been pretty important to me—especially where **my life** is concerned. (Take note—this issue comes up a number of times throughout this book and will, most likely, come up while you are struggling through this diagnosis.)

I went to see Dr. Dube on a Friday. Not seeming terribly concerned, she wrote the prescription for the mammogram and diagnostic ultrasound. The following Tuesday I went to my scheduled ultrasound appointment—with prescription in hand. Two days later, I returned to the hospital to pick up a copy of my x-rays and the diagnostic report for my surgeon, who wanted to review them during my appointment the next day.

I couldn't wait to read the radiologist's report. As I walked to my car with the sealed envelope, I could barely contain myself. As soon as I got into the car, I opened it. Not only was I surprised, but relieved by what I read (keep in mind that I *showed* the technician the cyst on my right breast and she *placed a marker on the area*).

MAMMOGRAM: Negative.

ULTRASOUND: Shows a cluster of cysts. No follow-up necessary.

Really??!! That's great!!

I immediately called Dr. Dube from my cell phone and left a message about the report, asking if I should cancel my surgeon's appointment. She called back a few hours later and said: "No, keep the appointment and let the surgeon have a look at it". (This is one of the first of what I have come to believe as 'Divine Interventions').

The next day, I went to see Dr. Willard, a female surgeon who was referred to me by my friend, Diana (...my second Divine Intervention). Diana wants nothing to do with hospitals, doctors and medicine (they actually make her nervous), but she does her research before diving into anything and always finds the best value for her money. Actually, Diana had discovered a cyst in her breast only three months before and had gone to Dr. Willard for the biopsy—which was negative. She was absolutely impressed by the doctor's personality, warmth and up-front attitude.

I found Dr. Willard to be everything Diana described...and more. Dr. Willard was also brash, very direct and above all—worthy of my trust and respect. We bonded instantly! At the end of my appointment, Dr. Willard suggested that I "just go ahead and have the cyst removed, biopsy it and be done with it". So we scheduled the outpatient surgery for the following Friday, November 7th.

Later that afternoon one of my very best friends called. Marge wanted to see if I could schedule a shopping day with her. For the past month, I had been helping her re-furnish and re-decorate her living room and she was anxious to have it finished in time for her birthday party on December 13th. We were working around her tight schedule and she only had one full day to shop and buy furniture before the day of the party. Even though it would be less than 24 hours after my surgery, I agreed to her picking me up the following Saturday to do some serious shopping.

On the day of my scheduled cyst removal, another friend, Trish, escorted me to the outpatient surgery department. My surgery was scheduled for 11:00am and would only take about 45 minutes. Not really concerned about the surgery or the results, I just wanted to get it over with.

The registration and the pre-op process went smoothly, including only one stick for my I.V. The nurse handed me a magic marker and had me write on my right breast "YES", which must be the result of several lawsuits relating to doctors who have removed the wrong arm or leg and operated on the wrong side of the heart, the brain, etc. *This made me proud that I was in healthcare???*

Anyway, I found it interesting that the nurse in the pre-op room, the nurse anesthetist, the anesthesiologist *and* the operating room nurse—immediately after introducing themselves—all asked me the same question. When I was asked for the fifth time "What did you have for breakfast?" (A trick question—since I was not allowed *anything* after midnight) I answered, "A BIG steak, 2 eggs over-easy and hash browns!!" At that point, they gave me the pre-op med and I went into la-la land.

What seemed like minutes later, I woke up with a small bandage on the right side of my right breast—which was right—I mean correct...and I was a little woozy from the anesthesia. Trish drove me home; I took a pain pill and slept through the night.

The next morning, Marge called to be sure that I was feeling up to a day of shopping. I looked down and checked my dressing—which was dry and intact. I didn't seem to be in any pain, so, I said, "Come on over. As long as I don't have to carry anything, or push open any heavy doors, I will be fine."

Believe it or not, we shopped from 10am until 6pm! It was relatively easy to pick out the *things that I wanted* and *Marge paid for.* I think my next career will be Interior Design. And...it's not everyone who can shop for 8 hours the day after surgery!

Over the next few days, I gave little thought to the biopsy results. I was quite sure that it was only a benign fatty cyst (just as my mother had when she was younger)...so I was not worried.

My thoughts were on two upcoming job interviews that I had scheduled for the following week. When my position was eliminated in March, I never believed it would be so difficult to find a job...but the country was in a panic with the war starting in Iraq. At this point, going to the gym everyday was a highlight in my life. After eight months of unemployment, I was looking forward to getting back to work.

On Tuesday morning, November 11th, as I was getting ready to go to the gym, the phone rang. It was Dr. Willard calling with the results of the biopsy. "I am sorry to tell you that the **results of the biopsy show breast cancer"**...

2. Hearing the Diagnosis

'You never know how brave you can be until it's your turn to be brave' —Author unknown

> **(Journal entry)** Tuesday, 11/11/03
> ...and then I had cancer.
> Today I got the results of the pathology report from my cyst that was removed on Friday. Dr. Willard had "that tone" in her voice and I knew before she even said the words. I caught bits and pieces of things that she said, but my brain just could not wrap itself around the words: Breast Cancer.

Breast Cancer. Cancer. The Big "C"...Really? She said I had **breast cancer**. *I can't believe it!*

I can't have cancer. I do have cancer; Dr. Willard read the pathology report. Maybe it's not my report. Maybe they mixed up my report with someone else's. I just read something in the newspaper about that happening last week. It happens. Oh yes, I also saw a story on 20/20 about a women who was misdiagnosed! She had her breast removed and she didn't even HAVE cancer! Dr. Willard said I should come in tomorrow to discuss the treatment options, so I am going to ask to see the pathology report. How could I have cancer????

Of course, the first stage of grief is "Shock and Denial".

Right after Dr. Willard's call, I didn't know what to do. In a daze, I went to the gym. During my workout, all I could think about was Dr. Willard's call...

Breast cancer? Who can I talk to about it? Who do I know that has breast cancer? No one that I can think of. Wait a minute...there was the local TV anchor woman who had it a few years ago...maybe I can call her. Yeah right, call her and say, "Hi Wendy...I remember watching TV a few years ago when you announced that you had breast cancer. Can we talk some time, because I was just diagnosed?" Oh right—I don't think so! Besides, I wouldn't even know how to get in touch with her. Hm-m-m...I wonder if she has an email address. Great...I am already starting to lose it.

I cut my workout short because I had to talk to someone. *The first person I must tell is Kelly.* I knew my daughter wouldn't take it well—the news would only serve to remind her of her father, who had died ten years earlier of lung cancer.

As I was packing up to leave, I decided to walk down and see Kelly, who lived about three blocks from the gym. I needed the fresh air, as well as the time to decide how I was going to break the news. When I got to her house, she wasn't there; so I walked back to the gym parking lot and began the drive home. On the way home, I felt the desperate need to share my diagnosis with someone, but felt strongly that Kelly had to be the first one I told. I tried her cell phone...no answer. *Where is she?!!!*

About two blocks from home, I noticed my daughter's car, at her best friend Michelle's house. *Thank you God!*

I did a quick right turn onto her street and as I pulled into the driveway, I saw Michelle and Kelly chatting on the sidewalk, apparently just finishing a long run. They were both surprised to see me and each came up to give me a big, sweaty hug.

As I squeezed her tight, I looked at Kelly and said, "I have something to tell you". She looked up at me and asked if I got the test results back from the surgeon. I nodded, with tears in my eyes. She immediately sensed my answer and started to cry hysterically.

Michelle looked quizzically at both of us and kept asking, "What's the matter...what's the matter?" I broke the news as we walked into the house with Kelly clinging to me and crying with hiccupping sobs.

Kelly's father died of lung cancer at the age of 45 when she was a senior in high school. Over the years since his death, her grief for him has sporadically risen to the surface. As I knew it would, this news created an emotional volcano with her feelings just spewing forth. "WHY?" she asked angrily. "Why is this happening to ME? First, my dad and now you! This isn't fair!!!" She sobbed as I held her close.

I looked into Kelly's eyes. "First of all," I said, "This isn't just happening to you. It's happening to me, too, and we are going to deal with it. Secondly, don't put me in the grave—breast cancer is one of the most treatable cancers there is, and I found this very early". Then, I shared as much information as I could remember from what Dr. Willard had told me on the phone that morning.

Still sobbing, my daughter looked at me as if she wasn't sure she should trust what I was saying. I told her that Dr. Willard wanted me to go to her office the next day, so that she could explain the pathology report and give me some details about treatment options. I asked her if she wanted to accompany me to the appointment. Tearfully, she nodded yes.

Kelly wanted to stay with her friend for awhile, probably wanting to share her feelings and talk...the way that only friends can.

I drove home alone and then made the next call—to my parents. My mother answered the phone and I blurted out the news. She responded as I knew she would—strong and supportive. I have always known that I got my stoic personality from my mom. Insisting that I would "come through this with flying colors", she emphasized that I was "a strong woman who would manage the treatment without problems." She went on to tell me that her hairdresser had breast cancer several years before and described how well she was doing. Then, she asked if I wanted to talk to my father.

My father, who had been diagnosed with prostate cancer about a year before, got on the phone.

"Well, Dad", I started, when he asked what was going on, "I have joined your club".

"What club?" He asked.

"The cancer club", I said. He immediately got quiet.

My big, strong father, who retired from a forty-year career in construction, got very emotional. He said he was so sorry to hear this kind of news and wished that I didn't have to go through it.

"I know", I responded, "but if we had to have cancer, you and I ended up with two of the most treatable ones."

I was trying to make him feel better—while I was still trying to convince myself that this was not a bad dream.

After getting off the phone with my parents, I went to my computer. I responded to an earlier email sent from an out-of-town friend who was writing to ask about my surgery and the results of the biopsy. Wendy had worked for two years selling a product that treated breast cancer and I needed her input on the information that Dr. Willard had given me (or at least THOUGHT I had been given).

I replied to Wendy's email.

Sent: Tuesday, November 11, 2003 11:53 am
Subject: Re: Recovering?
I got "the call" this morning and just finished telling Kelly. They found cancer---grade III. I have to go to the doc tomorrow morning to discuss the options. Will keep you informed. Definitely keep the prayers going.
Carla

Later that afternoon, the phone calls began and continued throughout the day—back and forth among friends who were asking about my biopsy...Marge, Diana, Trish and Barb. Every time I told some one the results, I got the same reaction: Shock and disbelief.

When I finally spoke to Wendy, I told her some of the details and apparently mentioned that I had Stage 3 breast cancer. Her overreaction startled me and she began to zing questions at me. "What are the margins? What is your ER/PR? Have they done a sentinel node biopsy?" I didn't have a clue what she was talking about.

As we were talking, her cell phone started cutting out and I could only hear every couple of words..."Her too...ductile...nodes". I totally lost the phone connection with Wendy. As I tried to redial, my phone rang again. It was Marge, calling to say that she was leaving work early and coming over to my house to be with me. She would be at my house about 5:00pm.

What Marge didn't know was that I had a date that evening and had to leave my house at 7pm. With this in mind, I hopped into the shower, got dressed, put some dinner in the oven and went to check my emails. I noticed that Wendy had written back.

Sent: Tuesday, November 11, 2003 5:29 pm

Carla —I'm sorry about my phone cutting out. I just read your original message after writing this and before sending it. Your note says GRADE III not STAGE 3! That is an important distinction! If the lump was only 2 cm—that is very early!!!!

There are several important questions you need to ask your doctor:

1. Is it ductile or lobular?
2. What is the hormonal status?
3. What is the 'HER' status?
4. Size of the lump removed
5. Status of the margins
6. Did they do a sentinel node mapping and if not why not?
   If they did not, then do they know the status of the nodes?

It is really doubtful that they could "stage" you without knowing the answer to several of these questions or without a CT scan. I have a feeling they were talking about the "grade" of the tumor or "how the cells look".

If you would like, I can ask about a good breast cancer oncologist in Orlando for you. You know I will help you in any way I can. I'll try and call you later tonight or tomorrow.

Thinking of You, Wendy

*Oops...I think I made a BIG-G-G mistake! I am so confused about this new information, that I must have told everyone that I had STAGE 3 breast cancer. Well, maybe not everyone, maybe only Wendy. Gosh, I have been in such a fog, I can't really remember **what I said** to anyone.*

I ran downstairs and started putting on my make-up. The door bell rang. As I opened the door, Marge stepped in, grabbed me and gave me a huge hug, choking on her emotions.

"I can't believe it", she said. I thought she was going to cry.

"I know", I answered without emotion.

At this point, I had been telling the story over and over and just didn't know if I could have another conversation about this today. I was feeling drained and distant.

I invited her to sit on the chair in my bedroom while I finished putting on my make-up.

"I have a date tonight", I said as I was drawing on my eye liner.

"What? You're going on a date?!!!" she asked with surprise.

"Well, yes. I made the date last week." I explained.

"Why don't you cancel?" She was serious.

"No!" I said emphatically. "I only met him a few weeks ago. What am I going to say? I have breast cancer, so I can't go out with you?"

"I don't feel any different than I did yesterday, when I didn't know I had cancer. No, I am NOT going to cancel!" I was getting a little agitated.

I didn't want to be rude, but while having this conversation, I was already formulating my defense against this disease. I knew that I didn't want to be treated any differently—or live my life any differently, just because cancer had entered into it. I guess I was consciously making one of my first choices. I was going on the date and Marge was going home after we had a bite to eat.

"Did I tell **you** that I had Stage 3 cancer?" I asked tentatively.

"Yes," she responded tearfully. "My mother had Stage 3 cancer when she was first diagnosed and she had a horrible attitude...and I watched her die—I am NOT going to let you do that!!" She started to cry.

"Oh my God, Marge," I confessed, "I think I may have made a mistake, I think Dr. Willard may have said **GRADE** III, not **STAGE** 3. I am so confused. Wendy says that they couldn't have staged my cancer yet...until a few other tests are done."

Somewhat relieved and ready to move onto another subject, we sat and ate some very dry, overcooked chicken, which I cut up over a salad. I then shooed Marge out the door at 6:55pm; got in the car and drove to meet my date at the movie theater.

We saw "Love Actually"—a very cute movie that had me laughing out loud, taking my mind off the fact that I had just been diagnosed with cancer that very morning.

After the movie, Phil and I stopped for a glass of wine and he asked me if I had heard from the doctor.

"No," I lied, "I tried to call today, but the office was closed. The answering service said the office was flooded over the weekend, due to a broken water pipe. *(true story!)* I will probably hear something tomorrow."

We had only been dating about three weeks and I wasn't ready for Phil to know about the cancer.

Later that evening, we said our good-byes and I got in the car to drive home. All of a sudden it HIT me—I have cancer!! And the tears started. I cried the whole way home and once I got inside the house, I began to realize the significance of the situation. Then I really started to cry...with a deep, soulful moan. I think it was the most sorrowful cry that I have ever had in my entire life. As I look back on that night, I understand how important it was to let go of all the emotion that had built up throughout the day.

I got into bed that night and after turning out the light, I screamed to the darkness: "I CAN NOT BELIEVE THIS!!!" I cried for hours—until I was all cried out. Emotionally exhausted, I finally fell asleep.

The next morning, Kelly and I went to see Dr. Willard, who carefully reviewed the pathology report with both of us. The doctor was very reassuring and repeated much of the information that she had given me the day before and that I had shared with Kelly. During the discussion, I pulled out Wendy's printed email and got answers to her questions:
1. Intraductile/Invasive comedo cell
2. ER-low-weakly positive / PR-negative
3. Positive
4. 1 cm
5. Not clear—lateral – intraductile
6. No—will schedule the sentinel node biopsy with next surgery

Dr. Willard outlined several options for treating the malignancy. Even though the tumor was small, the positive HER2 Neu and the comedo cell indicated an aggressive cancer. Because the margins were not clear, she would definitely have to go in again and remove another piece of tissue in hopes of getting a clear margin (meaning that there are no cancer cells along the edge of the tissue). That was option #1 and was called a "breast-saving procedure".

Option #2 was a single mastectomy (removal of the entire right breast) and Option #3 was a bilateral mastectomy (removal of both breasts), with the possibility of immediate reconstruction (inserting expanders for implants).

While discussing the options with Dr. Willard, I got the feeling that she was "leaning" toward a bilateral mastectomy, but she wanted me to talk with the oncologist before making any decision. She referred me to Dr. David Molthrop, an oncologist who, she said, was similar in personality to me. She emphasized that Dr. Molthrop was direct and would "tell it like it is"; that "he was research-oriented and kept up with all of the latest treatments". Dr. Willard then phoned Dr. Molthrop and talked him into squeezing me in for an appointment the next day.

During the meeting, Kelly asked a lot of questions and seemed to have a sense of relief when it was over. I knew that including her on this appointment was very important. If I had gone alone and then given her the information afterwards, she may have felt that I was holding something back—which would have caused her undue stress and anxiety.

Kelly was disappointed that she could not accompany me to the appointment with Dr. Molthrop. My daughter is a professional equestrian who shuttles between Orlando and the West Palm area to train horses and provide riding instruction. She had lessons scheduled the next day and would not be available to go with me to see the oncologist. However, several friends had already offered to help out and do "whatever I needed".

Marge, who is also a nurse, offered to go and "listen" to what the doctor had to say. I later realized that this was another Divine Intervention—because no matter how much medical education one might have, when diagnosed with cancer, you become "the patient" and it's impossible to digest everything the doctor says. *It is extremely important to have someone accompany you to your medical appointments. If at all possible, take someone who has some basic medical knowledge and isn't afraid to ask questions. Taking notes is also a good idea!*

While talking to Dr. Molthrop the next day, Marge and I both got the strong impression that he was "leaning" toward my having a breast conservation procedure, a sentinel node biopsy and then, if the cancer had progressed to the lymph nodes, a regimen of chemotherapy. I left feeling confused and unsure of what to do.

Two different doctors...two different opinions. Both agreed, though, that the decision was up to me as to how my treatment would proceed. Both physicians said that I had the CONTROL. But I wasn't sure that I wanted it, nor was I sure that I could handle it. So, I prayed that I would make the right decision.

That evening, I called my parents and about six friends, including Sandy Donnan, who I only see about once a year. Regretfully, I had forgotten that Sandy, too, had experienced breast cancer a few years ago. Our conversation and her advice was another Divine Intervention, as she said the words I needed to hear. "Everything is as it should be", she said in a comforting voice. "You will come out of this a *better person*...just surrender to God and He will take care of you."

Later, I wrote in my journal about my initial decision to go along with Dr. Molthrop's outlook on the breast conservation procedure. I felt that this procedure would buy me a little time, while waiting to see what the second pathology report showed.

Mentally, I compared the decision process to crossing a river on stepping stones...you have to get your footing on one stone before choosing the placement of your other foot. However, I was finding it to be a challenge just to get my foot on that *first* stone.

3. Making the Decision

'The man who insists upon seeing with perfect clearness before he decides, never decides'. —Henri Frederic Amiel

I have been blessed with having many friends in my life. Once or twice a year, I spend time with one particular group of women, all of whom share strong emotional and spiritual bonds. Every time we get together, we express amazement at the almost thirty years that we have known each other and the memories we have created.

Because of our busy agendas and hectic lives, it is always difficult to coordinate a weekend that fits everyone's schedule. However, long ago, we realized that if we look forward about six months, we can find a weekend that hasn't been filled and we all block it out on our calendars with indelible ink!

It seems that no matter when we get together, one of us has a serious, life-changing issue that requires the counsel and support that this group provides. The love that we share for each other has been proven over and over again as this healing group turns tears into laughter, sadness into joy and fear into strength.

So it was truly another Divine Intervention when, three days after I was diagnosed, a weekend had been scheduled with this wonderful group of women...all of us knowing that *I was the one* who would be embraced and supported throughout this weekend.

> **(Journal entry)** Friday, 11/14/03
> Marge came over and packed me into her car for our semi-annual trek up to High Springs to celebrate "WWWW: Wild Women's Weekend in the Woods." Linda was ready when we arrived at her workplace. She hoisted suitcase, cooler and pillows into the trunk and we all settled in for the 2 ½ hour drive to Pat's cabin on the Santa Fe River. Pat was anxiously waiting for us when we arrived at 5:30pm.

We dragged our luggage and pillows up the stairs to the porch and let them sit inside the door of the cabin as we all, in turn, embraced Pat with a big, warm hug. The next thing I did was pour myself a glass of wine as Linda started pulling chicken, mushrooms, herbs and rice from her cooler. She had volunteered to prepare the first gourmet meal of the weekend.

After a few minutes of relaxation, Marge and I started a friendly argument over who was going to get the bedroom and who was going to sleep on the sofa bed. I insisted that I should get the bedroom.

"Why should you get the bedroom?" Marge asked. "You had it the last time we were here."

"I know...but...I have cancer." I pouted.

"OH, so you're going to pull the cancer card!!!" She acted astonished. At that point, we all laughed hysterically and the tone was set for the weekend.

The conversation flowed (as did the wine); the food was fabulous and my friends were as comforting as a warm and snuggly robe. After dinner, we were sitting around the fireplace and Pat went into her bedroom. She came out with a gift that she had bought earlier that day. Without her reading glasses on, she kept trying to remove the 'price tag' (which was really a sticker that said "Squeeze Me"). When we realized what she was doing, we couldn't stop laughing because each time she tried to pull off the sticker, a recording of "Jesus Loves Me" continued to play!

I named the soft, cuddly, stuffed angel "Jackie" after a friend of ours who died of cancer several years before—a beloved member of the WWWW group, who I really felt was there in spirit with us that night.

The next day, our plan was to relax in the morning and then go into Gainesville for a daytime Art Show and evening Jazz concert. After cleaning up the breakfast dishes, Marge and I went out on the porch to check the weather. Taking a deep breath and inhaling the fresh air, she commented on how relaxing it was to "listen to the rush of the flowing river". As we stood there soaking in the peacefulness of the moment, we suddenly realized we were listening to the *flowing outburst from Pat's water tank* that was in a shed a few yards away!

Needless to say, the moment of peace and relaxation was gone and a plumber had to be found...on the weekend, no less! Apparently within this small community of seasonal residents, things like this happen all the time, so the plumber (and his son) came and quickly replaced the tank. After about two hours, everything was back to normal and we loaded the car with our picnic baskets and blankets and headed to Gainesville. We spent a few hours enjoying the art, along with the clear blue skies and warm sunshine. Later, we found a spot to lay our blankets and we listened to some fabulous live jazz from Mindi Abair, Greg Karukas and Jonathan Butler.

By 11pm, the concert was over and we drove back to the cabin. Prior to retiring for the night, Linda gave me a big hug and presented me with a beautiful glass paperweight she had bought earlier from one of the artists. She said that while admiring the piece, she knew that it was meant for me. I gratefully accepted the gift. It reminded me of a breast with sparkling bubbles inside...very symbolic.

On Sunday morning, the sun was shining through the windows, waking me at about 7:15am. This was unusual for me since I had been sleeping until 9am for the past eight months of unemployment. None of my friends were awake yet, so I rolled over and fell back to sleep. When I opened my eyes at 9:15am, the house was still quiet. Unable to sleep any longer, I got up and sat on the side of the bed. Taking advantage of the quiet morning, I began a prayerful meditation, focusing on my healing process and surrendering to God the outcome of this ordeal.

Twenty minutes later, no one in the cabin was stirring, so I decided to go out and enjoy the morning. After getting dressed and walking out to the end of the property, I sat down on a huge, warm rock in a sunny spot by the river. My thoughts began to drift to the upcoming months, not knowing what the future held for me. On some level, I was aware that I was creating a memory for future use—the cool river water flowing lazily, carrying away the leaves that were dropping from the trees, one by one. As the sun was kissing my face, I could feel its healing power; and the breeze shivering through the trees was alerting me to the fact that my angels surrounded me. A dragonfly lit near my toes and a butterfly skimmed across my path. As I sat there, I had a sense of peace, knowing that everything would work out for me.

I slowly sauntered back to the cabin only to find out that Marge and Linda were still sleeping. Pat was awake and dressed and had just stepped out onto the porch, preparing to join me down by the river. It was a gorgeous day...the sky was a glorious azean blue, the sun was shining brightly and there was a cool breeze...and we needed to get out and enjoy it! A plan was devised to get the others up. Pat started to brew the coffee while I noisily began making breakfast. *It is almost 11:00am and time for these ladies to rise and shine!!!* My friends were not happy about my banging the dishes, pots and pans, but they *were* up to the task of eating a hearty breakfast.

After a quick clean-up of the breakfast dishes, we went for a walk down the dusty country road that flanks the river properties. We all experienced the serenity of the moment and expressed our appreciation for the kinship we had shared over the years. As we strolled past fields of fresh green grass, huge oak trees with Spanish moss hanging from the boughs, verdant pastures with cows and horses and goats—we were creating another memory...it was like walking through heaven.

I was glad that my friends felt comfortable talking about my diagnosis. They asked if I had decided what I would do next. Sharing my decision that I was going the route of breast conservation, I told them my plan was to call Dr. Willard the next morning so that her staff could schedule the surgery.

On the way back to the cabin, Pat, who is a certified trainer in Healing Touch Therapy[1], suggested that the group perform a healing touch session prior to our leaving for home. *What a warm and nurturing sensation it was to experience the healing energy of these three people who love me and want me to be well.* It is Divine Intervention that these ladies are in my life.

The drive home was quiet as we were all relaxed from the weekend and even with the stress of the diagnosis and the decision about the next surgery, the time that I spent with these three wonderful women resulted in a feeling of peace about my upcoming journey.

The next morning, I was ready to share the information about my diagnosis with my dear friend who lives in Tucson. I sent Beth my "Cancer Announcement":

> Date: 11/17/03
> Subject: It's always Something...
> Hi Beth~ No job yet (it's been eight months!)...and last week I had a cyst removed from my right breast—which turned out to be malignant. I am seeing the surgeon this morning to plan for a second surgery and then will meet with the oncologist for a treatment plan. I am sorry to tell you this over an email, but I have been dealing with this for a week and have been on the phone every night since last Tuesday (when I was given the news). I spent the weekend in a cabin on the Santa Fe River with three of my very dear friends—a very timely gathering, as they are very spiritual and nurturing women.

I had two great interviews last week—can you believe it? Please
just keep me in your prayers, as I know you will.
Love you, Carla

After sending the email, I got into the shower to prepare for
my 10:00am appointment with Dr. Willard. As I was readjusting
my shower nozzle, I looked at the plastic information sheet that
was hanging there. Staring back at me was the "Monthly Breast
Self-Examination" instructions—which I use as a reminder to
check for lumps while in the shower. As I palpated the healing
incision on my right breast, I decided to check for lumps on my
left breast. Deep down under the left nipple, I thought I felt
another cyst. *I couldn't believe it!* With my fibrocystic breasts, it
was so difficult to determine what I was feeling. But, I would
definitely show Dr. Willard when I met with her later that
morning.

I arrived at Dr. Willard's office right on time. She was with
another patient but her nurse Susie came out to say hello.
Although she is probably in her late 60's, Susie has more energy
than most people who are thirty years her junior. Six years ago,
Susie had breast cancer and had decided on a single
mastectomy; and it is through this experience—to say nothing
of her bubbly personality—that she creates an instant bond
with her patients.

We talked about my diagnosis and discussed my decision to
have the breast conservation surgery. Susie was very supportive
and said that everyone who has breast cancer needs to make
the decision that is best for them. At that moment, however, I
was still unsure as to whether or not this was the right decision.

Susie escorted me to an exam room where I told her about
the second lump I felt that morning in the shower. She
suggested that the doctor might want to biopsy it and went to
talk with Dr. Willard. Sure enough, when Dr. Willard came in,
she requested a core biopsy needle from Susie, so that she could
get some tissue from the cyst that she, too, was able to locate
just beneath my nipple. Two shots of xylocaine and five minutes
later, Dr. Willard put a piece of tissue into a bottle to send over
to the lab.

As Dr. Willard was applying a band-aid to the area where she
had inserted the needle, she advised me to "ice the area" as soon
as I got home. Since I had planned to leave the office and do a
little shopping for Marge's living room, I asked Susie to make an
ice pack out of a rubber glove, which I squeezed into the left side
of my bra. Now I was really lop-sided, so I asked for a few paper

towels and stuffed them into the right side of my bra. After all of that, I could hardly button my blouse and I walked out of the office looking like Dolly Parton!!

The next morning, I was getting dressed to go to the gym and I got a phone call from Dr. Willard, giving me the results of the biopsy that was taken from my left breast. I held my breath as she told me the news. The pathology was benign. *Thank you, Lord!*

She also informed me that my surgery was scheduled for the following Monday. *So, this is starting out to be a good day.* I felt a welcomed sense of calm.

After a quick dinner that evening, I got on the computer to do some research about breast conservation vs. mastectomies. Not surprisingly, I found tons of information. Wanting to understand—without being overwhelmed—about the most current treatments, I focused on articles that were written by research-oriented cancer institutions and pharmaceutical manufacturers of breast cancer treatments. I printed out lots of material on ductile and invasive cancer and began trying to get a handle on what 'HER2Neu' is all about.

I felt compelled to learn as much as possible about what was growing inside me in an effort to make the best decision for my own treatment. After an hour or so on the computer, I received several calls from my friends. The last call that night was from my friend, Barb.

Several months prior to my diagnosis, Barb was diagnosed with Stage 0 breast cancer and had been through thirty daily radiation treatments. When I was first diagnosed, she provided me with an October issue of the CURE magazine which featured exclusive articles on Breast Cancer, treatments, survivors, etc.

"Have you decided what you are going to do yet?" Barb asked. Of all my friends, Barb certainly had the most up-to-date knowledge about breast cancer.

"I think I am going ahead with the quadrantectomy, so they can clear the margins." I said, hesitantly.

"Really?" She sounded surprised. "If it were me, I would do the most drastic thing I could do to get rid of it!" she said without taking a breath.

That really stunned me—and I was pissed! I could not believe that in a two minute conversation, Barbara had made me question my decision—AGAIN!

I was so angry that I lied and said that my phone was beeping, indicating that I had another call. Shaking my head I hung up the phone, not believing that the decision I had been *so sure of* was now going to be re-evaluated.

As I lay in bed that night, I began to re-visit my conversation with Barbara. *Is she right? Should I seriously consider having the bilateral mastectomies? I can't believe how I am "flip-flopping" with my decision about surgery. MY DECISION WAS MADE...AND NOW SHE HAS ME RETHINKING IT! I wish someone would just tell me what to do!*

After a fitful sleep, I got up early and went into the bathroom. I stared at myself in the mirror, trying to make sense of what I was dealing with. Finally, I threw my arms up into the air, asking for God's help in making the decision about the mastectomy. *I really don't know what to do. Please help me to know **what is right for me.** Help me, Lord...PLEASE help me!*

I washed my face, and got dressed, then drove to the gym. Another Divine Intervention! Wendy—the TV anchor woman to whom I wanted to talk when I was first diagnosed—was at the gym!!! She had just finished her workout and was getting ready to walk out the door, when a staff member (whom I had told about my cancer) stopped her and introduced us. When she mentioned that she is *never* in the gym this late, I got goose bumps—knowing this was a conversation I was meant to have.

Immediately, I delved into "my story" and started asking her questions about her breast cancer experience. She told me that she, too, had been diagnosed with ductile/invasive cancer—her sentinel node biopsy resulted in two 'questionable' lymph nodes. After some thorough research, she made the decision to have a single mastectomy. And when the doctor informed her that she had to have chemotherapy, she opted to go into a clinical trial.

This woman gave me so much hope when she told me that she *worked everyday* throughout her cancer treatment. Her only regret was that she wished she had made the decision to have a bilateral mastectomy. When I asked why, she said there were two reasons. First, her surgery left an obvious difference in the symmetry of her breasts—which was not really a *major* concern. More importantly she believed, it would have relieved some of the anxiety she feels every six months with each follow-up mammogram on her other breast.

With that conversation, and in conjunction with the research I had been doing, I suddenly felt sure that the right decision for me was to have a bilateral mastectomy. I truly felt that this serendipitous meeting was the result of my morning prayer...and I paused to say *Thank You, Lord.*

Thanking Wendy for her input, we said goodbye.

Then I thought: *"Yikes; I have to cancel my upcoming surgery!"* So, I immediately left the gym, called Dr. Willard's office and asked to speak with Susie.

"I know this is short notice and I'm sorry," I said, "But, I decided to have the bilateral mastectomies...and", I said without stopping to breathe, "To me, it doesn't make sense to have the surgery on Monday, and then undergo general anesthesia *a third time* to have the mastectomies. So I should cancel. Right? What do you think?"

Patiently, Susie said, "Carla, whatever you decide to do will be right for you. When Dr. Willard comes in, I will let her know your decision and she will give you a call to discuss it."

I spent the afternoon reading all about breast cancer in the October edition of the CURE magazine. I also went back online to do more research about the pros and cons of mastectomy. The information validated my decision, but also opened my eyes to the physical changes that go along with this surgery.

When Dr. Willard called, I was *certain* that I wanted to move forward with the mastectomies. I apologized for the inconvenience that I was causing; however, Dr. Willard said "It's perfectly fine for you to change your mind—and if you change it again, that will be okay too. I want you to be comfortable with your decision. We'll cancel Monday's surgery and make an appointment for you to see a plastic surgeon." *Gawd, I love this woman!!!*

That evening, my mother called. She and I discussed the mastectomy decision as I did later with Marge. They both supported my decision, calling it "wise". However, in my heart, I knew that they would support whatever I decided to do.

Three days went by and I received an email from Beth, who was my assistant head nurse eons ago. When I took maternity leave in 1976 and decided to stay home with Kelly, Beth was promoted to head nurse. I don't know if she has ever forgiven me for leaving her. We were a great team.

Over the past several years, I have traveled to the Southwest to visit her and we created some wonderful vacation memories in Sedona and the Grand Canyon. My sweet friend Beth is not the greatest at responding to emails, so I wasn't surprised when I got her "delayed" reaction.

> Date: 11/23/03
> Subject: Re: It's always Something...
> Oh, Carla...
> I just accessed my email for the first time in over a week due to computer problems—buried there amid over 90 mostly spam messages—was your heart-breaking news.
> I know you are one of those supremely strong women with a tightly-woven spiritual safety net, but I guess I never really cared for that saying "We only get what we can handle". I hope you realize you have been in my thoughts frequently...I've imagined many times the conversations we'd have once I finally connected with you...and I'm sorry I haven't made that physical connection for so many months. Ironically, I have a card on my desk that I picked out last week for you—to hold copies of the photos taken when we went to Sedona last year, with a 'remember when' message.
> You, of course, will now be in my thoughts every day many times. I'm glad you had that get-away on the Santa Fe, and I wish you quiet moments from the storm whenever they arise. I will come visit, also. I will have some PTO soon and would like to come see you. And if you say "yeah, sure..." I don't blame you a bit after that promise broken last spring...but all I can do is say "this is what I want" and see if the angels allow it! I will write/call/email soon...
> Much love to you, my friend...Beth

Within the first few weeks of diagnosis, I was beginning to get overwhelmed with the amount of attention that I was getting....and the cards! I couldn't believe the number of cards— get well cards, cards of encouragement, prayer cards, humorous cards, and serious cards. I was still trying to grasp the concept of my having cancer, when my sister sent me a pink card that actually had these words written on it: "The C-Word. Hard to say, Harder to Hear. When Cancer strikes, everything seems to get more difficult". I was amazed—Hallmark cards just aren't what they used to be!!! Of course, the words: Courage, Compassion, Concern and Care were all part of the verbiage, but, it was *this* card that punctuated the reality of my situation.

One day, I was reading a card from my parents. It was a beautiful card that said exactly what the sender wanted to say...straight from the heart. I started to cry because it touched me so deeply. While I was sobbing, my friend Kay called. I picked up the phone.

"What's the matter? Are you OK?" she asked in a panic.

"Yes, everything is fine." I said, "I was just reading a card that my parents sent and it touched me, that's all."

"Well, I'm coming over to see you. In fact, I'm on my way." Evidently, she wasn't going to take no for an answer.

About thirty minutes later, Kay rang the doorbell. As I opened the door, she said hello and immediately looked at my breasts. WHAT was THAT all about? Is EVERYONE going to look at me differently from now on? I decided to call her on it.

"Uh, Kay...do you realize you just looked at my breasts? What did you think they were going to look like—big giant masses of CANCER???" We both laughed and I smacked her on the arm as she walked into the house. Later, I showed her my tiny incision. This was the beginning of my trying to take the 'mystery' out of breast cancer.

After a nice long visit, Kay left and I took a huge breath. I was exhausted.

Due to the fact that I had been spending many of my days and evenings answering questions and explaining things over and over again, I decided to send an email to all of those who had been concerned about my health and the progress with my upcoming surgery. I would give all of them the details...at the same time.

> Date: 11/24/03
> Subject: Update
> Dear Friends and Family~
> I wanted to give you an update on what's going on and thank you from the bottom of my heart for all of the concern and support that you have expressed during the past two weeks. Believe it or not, there are over 30 people that I have been talking to these past couple of weeks and it will be impossible to update you all by phone, so I am taking advantage of this modern day convenience.
> Although it is still hard to believe, I am moving forward with the acceptance of this diagnosis, knowing that it is a process that I must go through as part of my life's path. I feel strongly that this experience will not only enhance my life, but will affect

yours—hopefully in a positive way—as well. If nothing more...at least I have you praying! I know there will be pain, both physical and emotional...but I am counting on our angels, saints and guardians to keep our spirits uplifted and keep the pain to a minimum.

I met with the surgeon this afternoon to discuss (again) my options and I have decided to have bilateral mastectomies with immediate reconstruction (perhaps 40-double D's??). I will meet with the plastic surgeon on December 4th to finalize details from his end and then coordinate scheduling the surgery with both docs and nuclear med (for a sentinel node biopsy—which determines if the cancer has spread to the lymph nodes). I made this decision, because of the type of cancer— intraductile/comedo invasive and because I don't want to go through the rest of my life being worried that every lump I feel could be another tumor.

I found out today that my surgeon, Sarah Willard MD, is not only trained in traditional Western medicine, but does energy work and healing, which goes along with my beliefs about 'complementary medicine'. Thanks to my friend, Jo, I am listening to pre-op meditation and affirmation tapes and will (upon anesthesia's approval) listen to a tape during surgery. However, Dr. Willard said she plays Steven Halpern's healing music CDs in the operating room.

Thank you again for your support and your prayers...keep praying...I truly believe in its power.
I love you all,
Carla

After sending the email, I felt good being able to put some of my thoughts on paper (or should I say onto the computer and thus into cyberspace). I enjoyed the fact that some relief may have been provided to those who were worried. I added a touch of humor, along with some spiritual guidance. With that email, I decided that all of my emails would contain a combination of those ingredients—and it would be my remedy for the pain that my family and friends would suffer, as they walked this journey with me.

As I began to receive the responses to my emails, I recognized that, not only would I teach my email group about breast cancer and my personal experience with it, but I would also learn from my family and friends. They would reveal to me their spiritual depth, along with their silly humor. But most of all, I would learn about the love and faith we shared with each other.

In this book, I will relate these responses, so that you may see the importance of reaching out to others for support. They are great examples of trusting that when you ask for help you will be provided with *exactly what you need... when you need it.*

Throughout these pages, you will notice how this happened to me. Call it what you will, but I continue to describe it as 'Divine Intervention'.

Dear Carla,

What a beautiful note! Have I told you how proud I am of you? Your strength and spirit and gusto all blow me away!

I hope you will keep the email that you sent and any others that chronicle this time that you are experiencing. It would be a beautiful journal of strength to share with others. And the stats are, I think, that one in four women will go through this. I, too, see this as a growing and learning time and the beginning of a whole new and glorious phase. I've heard more than one woman speak of it as a gift in her life. Strange how that works, isn't it?

I really didn't like the idea of you having your surgery while I was to be away today, so I am glad that you changed your surgery date.

Please plan on my driving you to and from surgery and/or anything else. I can and want to take off from work as much time as needed to be there for you, so just keep me in the loop as far as appointments go, okay?

By the way, haven't you ALWAYS been double-D?

Mucho love,

Trish

P.S. I wanted you to see my sister Suzy's response to your update...

Date: Tue, 02 Dec 2003
Subject: RE: Carla's Update
I can't get over Carla's attitude about all this. I didn't realize she was such a spiritual person. I'm so proud of her and can only hope that I could possibly be only half as upbeat (that's really not the right word, but I'm at a loss) if this happened to me.
I like her so much and am very hopeful that everything will be all right.
Tell her I'll keep her in my prayers.
Suzy

Dear Carla,
Thank you so much for including me in this group of friends.
You are on my mind and in my prayers daily. I am so glad that
you are looking forward, rather than being paralyzed by the
news. My prayer is for healing and for God's hand to be on you
and all who care for you. Know that I will continue to pray...and
that you are loved. I am so sorry that you have to go through
this. Olga

Carla,
Thank you for the update. Your surgeon sounds wonderful and
it appears that your support network is falling into place for
this most special and extremely important chapter of your life!
We are all there, loving and rooting for you.
Love you, Pat S.

Dearest Car:
What a beautiful way to lay it all out. The only part I am slightly
concerned about is the 40 double D's. Won't you be at risk for
frequently falling over forward? Or could it be that I am jealous?
I love you and send all my energy, shared faith and dark humor
to sustain you through this episode. I plan to visit at the end of
January or in February, but will wait to see when you are ready.
Always, Maur

My journal entries continued for a while longer...these were
private thoughts that, at the time, I didn't want to share with
others in my emails. But, I felt a need to express and keep a
copy of my early emotions:

(Journal Entry) Tuesday 12/02/03
Well, I could have stayed in bed ALL DAY—but, I listened to my
pre-surgery meditation and affirmation CD—then forced myself
to get up and dress for the gym.
I "stayed in my head" during the whole time that I was working
out. John, one of the gym staff, commented that it didn't look
like I "was into it today." He was so right. When I was on the
Cardio machine, I acknowledged my depressed feelings,
blessed them and asked them to leave.
I do feel "quiet" this afternoon, wondering if I am starting to
grieve the loss of my breasts. I still believe that it's the right
decision and will ultimately lead to my cure; however it will be
hard to say good bye to them.

One of the conscious decisions that I made early on, was that I would not "listen" to any negative comments about breast cancer...or surgery...or chemotherapy. This was going to be MY experience and I didn't want to hear about the horrible things that happened to other people who "went through something similar".

Sometimes people would want to tell me things that weren't even close to being similar to what I was about to experience...and I "cut them off at the pass".

With everything I was about to go through, I wanted to keep positive thoughts about the process and the outcome...and I didn't want any negative thinking to have an effect on that. I probably insulted some of my friends when I told them that I didn't want to hear their stories if they had even the slightest tone of negativity.

> Hi Carla,
> It was so good to see you again. Meant to drop you a quick note before now.. but have been really engrossed this week!!! Got Christmas decorating done, shopping completed, cards finished, and we had a great turkey day besides!!!!
> You are doing great with this...keep those positive thoughts.
> I have been thinking more about what I was trying to say at lunch the other day. What I realized after my surgery was how frustrating it was not having control over how things unfolded. It doesn't mean that I didn't deal with it and deal with it well...but it is just so easy to forget that, even though you may do every thing *right*...your body might have another path in mind for you. So...I really wasn't trying to interject a negative note...and I really believe that you are in a good state of mind.
> However, from working with people going through massive change, another thing I have learned over the years is that one of the most difficult things in going through changes are the surprises...so you may be more resilient if you expect the emotions and frustrations that are an inevitable part of this kind of process.
> You are doing so many things right...and we are all praying for you. Be sure to let me know when the surgery is scheduled. We will keep you in our hearts and in our prayers.
> Jo and Craig

Although I didn't realize at the time, Jo was predicting an emotional outcome that I would not feel for many, many months to come.

Instead of focusing on her advice about unexpected emotions and frustrations, I focused instead on the prayers.

Having been raised in a Catholic family, it is important to understand that, with a diagnosis of cancer, there is a lot of praying going on! In fact, anytime someone is in pain, undergoing diagnostic tests, getting ready for surgery, going through surgery, recovering from surgery, is pregnant, or is about to deliver a baby...(you get the picture?)—there is ALWAYS a patron saint that will help you through it. Catholics ask these saints to intervene, and pray to God, on our behalf.

Anyway, one night my mom called to check up on me, and we got into a conversation, pondering the patron saint of cancer and who that might be.

"I don't have a clue", I said to my mom.

"Well, I KNOW there is one...I think his name starts with a 'P'." She said emphatically.

"Well, I know that I haven't *ever heard* of a cancer saint." I said, just as emphatically.

"I am sure that either Ann or Janis knows who it is, because they have mentioned it to me before. I think his name starts with a 'P'", she repeated.

"Ok, mom, just let me know when you find out, because I really and truly, DEFINITELY need to ask him to pray for me."

The next day, I received two separate emails from each of my sisters, Ann and Janis, who "found" the patron saint of cancer and the prayer for patients with cancer. Ever since my diagnosis, I have been asking him to pray for me and women that I know who have also been diagnosed with breast cancer. For those who would like to do the same, here are two prayers:

A Prayer to St. Peregrine for Sick Relatives and Friends

O great St. Peregrine, you have been called "The Mighty"
and "The Wonder Worker" because of the numerous miracles
which you obtained from God
for those who have turned to you in their need.
For so many years, you bore in your own flesh this cancerous
disease that destroys the very fiber of our being.
You turned to God when the power of human beings could do
no more, and you were favored with the vision of Jesus
coming down from His cross to heal your affliction.
I now ask God to heal these sick persons
whom I entrust to you:

(here mention their names)
Aided by your powerful intercession, I shall sing with Mary a
hymn of gratitude to God for His great goodness and mercy.
Amen.

A Prayer to St. Peregrine for One Suffering from Cancer
Dear St. Peregrine, I need your help.
I feel so uncertain of my life right now.
This serious illness makes me long for a sign of God's love.
Help me to imitate your enduring faith when you faced
the ugliness of cancer and surgery.
Allow me to trust the Lord
the way you did in this moment of distress.
I want to be cured, but right now I ask God
for the strength to bear the cross in my life.
I seek the power to proclaim God's presence in my life
despite the hardship, anguish and fear I now experience.
O Glorious St. Peregrine, be an inspiration to me and
petitioner of those needed graces from our loving Father.
Amen.

Well, as moms always are...my Mom was right about St. 'P',
the patron saint of cancer. Just for good measure, she even sent
me a St. Peregrine medal!

Carla-
    Have you found out anything new concerning your surgery? I
wish it was over and you were on the mend. Today, I sent your
dad to the Post Office to mail your St. Peregrine medal and a
necklace with Our Lady of the Miraculous Medal; I hope they get
there by Thursday. We love you and are praying for you...and
we have half the members of St. Andrew's Church praying also.
Love you and hang in there!
Mom and Dad

Carla-
    Hello...how are you??? I can not imagine what you are going
through. Please know that my thoughts, prayers and lit candles
go out to you. Mom has kept me updated with all that is going
on. If there is anything...anything at all that I can do, please
don't hesitate to call. I love you and hope all goes well. I think
your decision to have the mastectomy as opposed to the
lumpectomy is a wise one. If you need a nurse to be with you
let me know, I will be there. Take care, Love-Your sis, Debi

Debi~

Thank you so much for your touching email. It is very generous for you to offer to be with me. Obviously, I have no idea what's in store and am grateful for all of the words of encouragement and support and offers to be of help. Maybe my lesson in this will be to ask for help...something I have always found difficult. I appreciate your prayers and know that they will provide me with whatever I need to get through this. I am praying that the timing of the surgery will allow me to enjoy our time together in North Carolina. Looking forward to seeing you and the family.

I love you, too. Carla

4. Taking Control (Yeah, Right)

'Today you can make your life significant and worthwhile. The present is yours to do with as you will.'
—Grenville Kleiser, American Writer

Dependent upon various factors, radiation therapy may be used as an adjunct to treat breast cancer. When radiation is required, there is usually a waiting period after the end of treatment before implants can be inserted to give the radiated tissue time to heal.

Since my cancer was caught early and the tumor was very small, my oncologist informed me that I did not need radiation therapy following my bilateral mastectomies. I was very happy about this news because I was hoping to have "immediate reconstruction". This means that after the breast surgeon performed the mastectomies, the plastic surgeon would then complete the first surgery by placing temporary saline expanders under the chest muscles in preparation for permanent breast implants.

I spent the next two weeks anxiously awaiting my appointment to see the plastic surgeon.

The night before my appointment, I stood in front of the full-length mirror, looking at my naked body. Focusing on my breasts, I began to reflect on their importance, both physically and emotionally. I thought about what they represented to me as a woman: Motherhood. Femininity. Sexuality. Intimacy.

Amazed that I had never before identified my breasts in such specific terms...it hit me like a ton of bricks! *Will I lose these precious gifts of womanhood following this surgery?*

I took the time to once again consider my options. *No...I thought...I have done my research and my decision is firm.* At that point, I prayed that my decisions were the right ones and placed my life and my future in the hands of a Higher Power. I trusted that I would be given the strength and the courage to deal with the physical changes that would soon take place.

The next day, I walked into the doctor's office for my consultation. Dr. Rotatori's reputation as one of the city's most respected and talented breast reconstruction surgeons, supported the confidence in my decision. I don't know what I expected; but when I met Dr. Rotatori, I found him to be a quiet and reserved physician who offered a calm and caring attitude toward my situation.

Dr. Rotatori sensed my nervousness as I asked a variety of questions. He could also see through my fear as I joked that he was the first person to ever take "pornographic pictures" of my breasts. He never cracked a smile.

Somehow, I felt he was showing his respect for me by letting me take the lead on how our physician-patient relationship would develop. He was very reassuring about my decision for the bilateral mastectomies and was sensitive to all my concerns. He even mentioned that he had seen three women in his office that very day, who were finishing up the last of the 3-phase process of their reconstructive surgeries.

When I asked if I could speak to one of them, Dr. Rotatori sent his nurse out to request permission from one of his patients. To my relief, a patient named Lorraine welcomed the opportunity to share her story with me.

The nurse escorted me to the exam room, where Lorraine was patiently waiting for insurance authorization for the "tattooing" of her areola, the last stage of her mastectomy reconstruction. Although, I thought I would just say hello and ask Lorraine a few questions, she instructed me to sit down. She then began to educate me about some of the events that I would soon come to experience. This gracious lady offered information, details and suggestions that I could *never* have found anywhere in my research.

Thirty minutes later I hugged Lorraine good-bye. And, for the first time, I felt completely satisfied that I had made the right decision, feeling perfectly comfortable in moving ahead with my surgical plan.

On the drive home, I began thinking about the upcoming surgery and how my parents and four siblings would react to my plan. My family has always been wonderfully supportive of each other and, although we are emotionally close, geographically we are thousands of miles apart. Even with our hectic work lives and crazy family schedules, we have made it a point to gather together at least every other year for Christmas. This year our extended family was planning a week-long reunion in a 10-bedroom house at the Outer Banks in North Carolina.

Reflecting on the fact that I would soon be sharing Christmas with my family and knowing that my friends could care for me post-operatively, I decided that there was no need for anyone to make the trip to Florida for my surgery—especially since the surgery date was so nebulous. However, I knew it would take some convincing for my parents not to attempt the drive from Pennsylvania.

My family is a continuing source of strength for me, particularly when handling difficult circumstances. My parents have provided me with core values and a solid faith that underscored my attempts to stay emotionally balanced while working through this treatment. My brother, Bill, who is the oldest, has always felt the burden of taking care of his "little sisters"—me and my three younger sisters, Ann, Janis and Debi.

As a result of the emotional roller coaster that Janis went through during her divorce several years ago, we have become quite close—and since we share the title of "single sister", we do whatever we can to promote the "fabulous-ness" of singledom!

We have traveled together and tend to get into trouble, no matter where we go. To avoid humiliation to any of our other family members, we have come up with monikers when we travel. Janis' name is 'Bunnie Ghirardelli' and mine is 'Mimi Godiva'. My sister, Ann, who is currently going through a divorce and will soon be joining the single sisterhood has been bestowed the name 'Cookie Valrhona'. As you can tell...we all love chocolate!

In addition to our chocolate monikers, we have decided that, since none of us look our age, we will never tell anyone the truth about how old we are (the Gabors have NOTHING on us!)

I had to laugh as all of these things went through my mind; as well as the thought that I just wanted to get this surgery over with—as soon as possible—so that my daughter and I could spend the holidays with my family.

The next morning, I prepared to send out a routine email to inform my family and friends of the latest plan and update in the saga of "Carla's Cancer experience". As I sat staring at the computer, I began thinking about my treatment and realized that—from beginning to end—my cancer treatment would take almost a full year.

God! How am I ever going to do this?

Recognizing that I would need alot of help throughout this experience, the importance of physical and emotional support became extremely apparent. If I hadn't had so many friends and family members available to me, I would have looked for a local cancer support group, either through the American Cancer Society or the hospital.

Not only did *I* need support, but those who loved me would need support, as well. Having spoken with several cancer survivors at the beginning of this journey, I was told that open communication and ongoing messages of strength, hope and joy *should be shared* among those who were worried about me and who had fears of their own. So...I decided to start my own support group—via email!

I was determined to turn this into an opportunity for education—sharing not only my physical experiences, but my emotional and spiritual experiences, as well. I expected that significant changes would occur in my life over the next year. And just as a caterpillar evolves into a butterfly, I felt strongly that I would come out of this experience a new and evolved person. The emails were entitled 'Metamorphosis'...

> Sent: Friday, December 05, 2003
> Subject: Metamorphosis - Part I
> *'The unendurable is the beginning of the curve of joy.'*
> —Djuna Barnes
>
> Well, I *wanted* to provide you with a surgery date; however, I will not have one until at least next Monday, as the two surgeons' offices are trying to coordinate a date with the hospital. The preliminary guess is that it will be sometime during the week of December 15th.
>
> Yesterday, I went to visit my plastic surgeon, Scott Rotatori, who introduced me to Lorraine, a 43 yr. old woman who had bilateral mastectomies in May. She was completing her final phase of the 3-stage procedure. Lorraine was kind enough to spend time with me talking about the surgery, the healing process and the stages of reconstruction.
>
> Yes, Lorraine was happy to show me her new and—might I say—VERY perky breasts. I have to say the surgeon is quite an artist. This "display" of creativity further eased my mind that the decision I have made is the right one for me. Lorraine assured me that I, too, would soon be sharing the ranks of the "Divine Secrets of the Ta Ta Sisterhood"! (So far, I have talked to about 4 women who have had breast cancer with mastectomies and all of them are most willing to show me their breasts! It's amazing!!!)
>
> I am still feeling great—having eliminated alcohol and sugar (my name is Carla Chesser and I am addicted to sugar) from my diet, I am taking some nutritional supplements to maximize my post surgery healing. I continue to work out at the gym daily,

listen to my meditative tapes and of course, pray for the best outcome possible.

Again, I must thank you for your calls, cards, prayers, mass cards, holy water, medals and your overwhelming offers of assistance. I would never wish this on anyone; however, it's great to know that the friends and family with whom I have surrounded myself in my lifetime are so wonderfully caring and supportive.

I will let you know *as soon as I know* when the surgery is scheduled...and then I will be calling upon you for the favors that you have so generously offered. (Uh-huh!)

In the meantime, The Breast Cancer website is having trouble getting enough people to click on it daily to meet their quota of donating at least one free mammogram a day to an underprivileged woman. It takes less than a minute to go to their site and click on "donating a free mammogram" (scroll down to the pink window in the middle). This doesn't cost you a thing. Their corporate sponsors/advertisers use the number of daily visits to donate mammograms in exchange for advertising. Here's the web site—pass it along to people you know   http://www.thebreastcancersite.com
I will talk to you soon.
Love, Carla

Carla:
You are sounding so good in your writings. I've thought about you so much, and attribute your great attitude and resiliency to the rest, revitalization and good living you've done this year, while you have been unemployed. I think you're just in a fantastic space and I continue to be awed by you!
Luv, Trish

I received the following from Barbara, who was the initiating factor in my decision change regarding lumpectomy vs. mastectomy.

Carla,
It sounds like everything is moving along. It's pretty amazing how women are willing to share their story and bare their breasts, isn't it? (I can tell you that plastic surgery, for whatever reason, has a tendency to do that to you!) Once, while waiting for a radiation treatment, I met a woman who was having some problems with her breast prosthesis. Never meeting me before, she asked me to help "straighten" her

breasts so they would look symmetrical. I was so astounded...but this disease has a way of bringing life into direct focus. It's a fight we all battle together as part of the sisterhood.

Will the reconstruction be a skin flap initially and then reconstruction at a later date? Since you opted for the double mastectomy, are you still doing chemo and radiation? Will I see you at Marge's party on the 13th? No drinking alcohol or eating sugar—was that of your choosing?

Keeping you in my prayers, Barbara

(As you read these emails, you will begin to see the educational need that we all have regarding breast cancer and its treatments.)

Three days later, my impatience got the best of me. I called Dr. Willard's office to ask if they had been able to schedule my surgery. Obviously, I wanted the surgery scheduled as soon as possible so that Kelly and I could make the trip to North Carolina for the Christmas holiday. Also, I was looking forward to Marge's big birthday bash to "show off" the fabulous room that I had spent so many hours redecorating.

As I was questioning Susie, she informed me that she had no information about my surgery, and Colleen—the scheduler—would not be in until the following morning.

A little annoyed, I told Susie that I was hoping to know something TODAY! Sensing my irritation, Susie kindly said that she would check on it and get back with me as soon as possible.

When I got off the phone, Kelly commented on my rudeness in expressing my frustrations with the nurse. I felt horrible! I realized that my continued efforts of trying to control events and timing were still at work here.

Knowing that I should not have taken out my disappointment on Susie, I went into my bedroom and threw up my arms in prayer, asking to place this issue in God's hands, knowing that HIS timing—not mine—was acceptable.

Later that afternoon, I decided to do a little shopping. I certainly did not feel the Christmas spirit, but definitely needed the diversion.

As I was driving home, my cell phone rang. It was Marilyn from Dr. Rotatori's office calling to tell me that they had a cancellation...and that she had scheduled me for surgery in two days! "Is that okay with you?" she asked.

"Are you kidding me?" I screamed. "It was exactly what I had been hoping for!" I was overjoyed!

It was then that I recalled one of the most important things that Lorraine had shared with me during our conversation in the plastic surgeon's office: *"Let your friends and family help you through this. You are going to need their help and they want to do things for you. Forget about your independent nature and let them."* Although I was reluctant, this advice would be valuable throughout my treatment experience. I couldn't wait to get home to start calling and emailing everyone with the news.

Having explained to my family that I *really* did not want them to make last minute travel plans to come for the surgery, I had to count on my daughter and my friends. With only two days advance notice, I needed to line up some help in caring for me post-operatively. So, I put out the request:

Sent: Monday, December 08, 2003 5:41 PM
Subject: Metamorphosis: Part II
Well gang...
AGAIN, my prayers have been answered! The doctors were looking at scheduling me for surgery some day next week, while I was hoping to have it this week. So, this morning, once again, I put it in the hands of the Lord and...the surgeon's office just called—someone else's surgery was cancelled and they have a slot open THIS WEDNESDAY, December 10th. So, I have to be at the hospital at 6:30am for an 8:30am appointment with the Nuclear Med department to place the wires/dye for the sentinel (lymph) node biopsy. My surgery will be around 1pm. I will probably stay in the hospital two days, with a PCA pump in hand.
Needless to say, the planning time is not what we all thought it would be, so I know that I am imposing on everyone's schedules regarding these particular dates.
Kelly's birthday is December 11th, Marge's big birthday bash is December 13th and the Baldwin's are having our bi-annual family Christmas reunion scheduled for December 21-28 in the Outer Banks, NC. I doubt that there would be any "convenient" time to have this surgery. All I know is that I want these cancer cells out of my body and the healing to begin ASAP. So, once again, I am requesting your prayers on the 10th, asking that the cells are contained in the breast and haven't gotten into the lymph nodes and that my healing time is as short as possible.

If any of you are available to be with me either during the hospitalization and/or the recuperation at home, I would appreciate knowing that.

WANTED: A number of caregivers who will provide assistance in getting a "lightweight" up in a chair and dressed. Will need help with meals and clean up. Comfortable accommodations are available: separate guest room and bath. Access to computer and high-speed internet. Continuous entertainment guaranteed with antics including loud snoring, my face without make-up, the inability to go to the bathroom by myself and calling for pain medicine. HBO and Showtime included.

Those who can help, give me a call. The others will have to wait to talk to me. HA!!!!

Love you all,

Carla (alias) "Mimi van Breastus"

As usual, my friends amazed me with their quick and supportive responses. With each email and phone call, I began to create a schedule of who was going to stay with me during surgery, recovery, and the two nights in the hospital. As a nurse, I know how important it is to have someone with you throughout a hospital stay, as an advocate for your care and treatment. (If the nurse is too busy to respond to your pressing the call button, it is nice to have a person who can get up and go out to the nurses' station and get the help you need.)

The schedule was filling up and everything was falling into place. *It was unbelievable!* In fact, I even made an EXCEL spreadsheet with names and phone numbers of all my local friends—along with a calendar of those who were scheduled to be with me throughout my hospital stay; who would drive me home on the day of discharge and those willing to care for me once I got home. Yes, once again, Carla was in CONTROL!!!

Hey LALALALALALA!!

I tried calling earlier using the number that was in my old phone and left a message. Did you get it or did I irritate some unsuspecting soul?

Wish I could come and be your nurse (well, at least a "go-fer")...but there's no way I can bail from here. I have no one to cover for me at the marina.

You are in my prayers LaLa, and I know that this is going to go well and that you're gonna get your ass up here to see me someday!!! XXXOOO helen

Carla:

It's a little late now, so I'll call ya tomorrow, but I can help WHENEVER! I am supposed to have a party here Friday night (about 34 people—mostly Fred's golfing buddies and wives, and a few folks from Errol). But of course I could and would cancel. Do you want someone there with you Wednesday morning while you are in between Nuclear Med and surgery??? OK, as I said—I'll call in the am!
Goodnight!
Sharon

Car~

You are unreal...the advertisement is quite appealing, but I am targeting the end of January to try and get down there. Does this mean you will make it to the Baldwin reunion?

I will surely be praying for you tomorrow, as I did last night at mass (Immaculate Conception). I know your strength and faith will see you through, and this will be behind you before we all know it.

I send my love ~Maur

Carla...

Good to hear the surgery is scheduled. I will let the Sisters know! I am in town and available and would be happy to help in anyway. Plug me in as you need me. I will try to call you this afternoon but I would imagine you are going to be swamped with calls.

Holding you in the light with full intention for your complete and speedy recovery.
Love, Sue

Hi Carla,

I will be thinking of you non-stop tomorrow and sending you not only prayers, but lots of positive energy...and so will Craig.

I am out of town for the rest of the week; I leave tomorrow morning. What do you have lined up so far? How long will you need someone to stay with you? Let me know how you are doing with the offers...Jo

Carla...Tried to connect via phone, you've got to be running around dealing with the last minute crush. I will be there on Thursday to sit with you after surgery.
We are all praying that you will be surrounded in Light.
Love, Sue

Carla-

Good luck. I hope all goes well and that the cancer cells are contained. My thoughts and prayers will be with you Wednesday. God and your angels will also be looking over you. I need to check my schedule and will let you know if I can get time off to come down to help out. Since the surgery has been moved up...are you coming to the Outer Banks for the family reunion to do your recuperating? Love you, Debi

The night before surgery, I was actually looking forward to the procedure. I just wanted to get it over with as soon as possible and let the healing begin. I also thought that the sooner I had the surgery the closer I would be to making my family reunion, which was almost two weeks away...*plenty of time to recover from the operation.*

Before leaving for the hospital the next morning, I did a quick check of my emails and was overwhelmed by messages of support, prayer and love:

Hi dear friend,

I went out to dinner tonight. Sorry it's too late to call you. As I go to bed you are on my mind and in my heart and prayers. May God be with you throughout tomorrow and keep you safe. I'll check on you during the day and will be with you in spirit every minute. I love you and am so blessed to have you in my life. Trish

Dear Aunt Carla,
I'm thinking about you. I hope that all goes well and that you have a quick recovery! Love, Erin

My thoughts and prayers are with you..........
love you, BRW

Carla:
My thoughts and prayers are with you. I just feel that you will do great and that the cancer will be contained. I am available anytime after Wednesday (12/17) in the afternoon and beyond. Even though it will be one week post surgery and you will probably feel that you may not need assistance, it would be wonderful to hang out with you, do some Healing Touch, cook, spend quiet time with you, whatever....Just let me know.
I love you, dear one.
Pat S.

5. Having the Surgery

'Life is an opportunity, benefit from it. Life is a beauty, admire it. Life is a dream, realize it. Life is a challenge, meet it. Life is a duty, complete it. Life is a game, play it. Life is a promise, fulfill it. Life is sorrow, overcome it. Life is a song, sing it. Life is a struggle, accept it. Life is a tragedy, confront it. Life is an adventure, dare it. Life is luck, make it. Life is life, fight for it!'
                                                        —Mother Teresa

I have so many fascinating friends and although I can only get together with some of them every few months, it is always with shared anticipation that we find a slot on our calendars to place us in a restaurant on the same date and the same time. Going back a few weeks—prior to my scheduled surgery—I met a couple of friends for lunch.

Sue, a gentle and spiritual woman, started her career in the Army as a Medic. She eventually became a Social Worker and was soon working to create programs related to the prevention and treatment of child abuse. Years later, she became the Vice President of a large hospital system and ran one of its hospitals. Finding the politics to be a source of frustration and unhappiness, Sue put a new spin on her life and completed her studies as a "Spiritual Counselor".

Jo has a doctorate in nursing and is an entrepreneur in the field of nursing—having written several books and educational programs focused on the integration of happiness and joy in the workplace. Her life's work is teaching others in the clinical field how to avoid "burn out" thus creating a sense of satisfaction in their work, rather than hopelessness in a career that is often filled with daily stresses.

Although I have never heard Jo speak to a group, I am sure she holds her audiences spellbound. She is an avid reader and can, at the drop of a hat, mention authors, books or tapes that are timely and integral to any conversation that we might have. Sue and I are continually amazed by this.

On the day of our scheduled lunch, we met at a favorite restaurant, and hugged each other as if we had not seen each other in months—which, of course, we hadn't!

After catching up on what was happening in each of our lives, Jo pulled a plastic bag out of her purse and handed it to me. Knowing that I was undergoing surgery, she gave me three books that I had not yet read and a packet holding two CDs, entitled "Successful Surgery"[2].

Fascinated, I began reading the inner flap of the packet which informed me that inside I would find an audio meditation program to prepare me for surgery. Apparently studies had been conducted at several well known University research centers, and using this program had resulted in enhanced recovery processes for patients who were undergoing surgery.

In the weeks prior to my surgery—each night for twenty minutes—I listened to the "Successful Surgery" guided imagery CDs. My mind and body began to anticipate a successful surgery experience, surrounded by protection and support with the body slowing down blood flow and speeding up its mending capacity. Along with the guided imagery were affirmations that would work to reduce pain and speed healing.

On the night before surgery, Kelly spent the night at my house. At 5:30am, the alarm rang and we hurried to get ready for our trip to the hospital. It was a cold morning, but I was in good spirits and absolutely ready for the procedure to begin.

We drove into the hospital garage and went directly to the Surgery admissions office. Shortly after my 6:30am arrival, the nurses had me out of my clothes and into a hospital gown. As they did prior to my cyst removal, the same questions were asked by everyone with whom I came in contact. "What is your name? Who is your doctor? What procedure are you having? When was the last time you ate?" The nurse gave me a surgical marker, so that I could mark both of my breasts with the words: "Yes", so there would be no mistaking that both of my breasts were to be removed. (Kelly wanted me to draw smiley faces on them, but I vetoed that idea.)

At about 8:30am, I was wheeled down to Nuclear Medicine, where the "node mapping" would take place. This procedure would help the surgeon locate the lymph nodes closest to the cancerous area in order to remove them and determine if the cancer had spread.

The staff was friendly and very precise and the mapping procedure was over in about 30 minutes. I was wheeled directly to the Pre-op holding area, where I waited while listening to my Healing CD music. My I.V. was started and I was feeling peaceful and relaxed, before remembering that I had forgotten to take out my contact lenses. The nurse had to call Kelly from the hospital cafeteria to bring my lens case and retrieve the contacts. After staying a few minutes and wishing me luck, Kelly kissed me and whispered in my ear, "I love you" and left for the waiting room.

Shortly after Kelly left, my favorite surgeon Dr. Willard strolled in, looked at me sideways and told me that "angels were all around" me. She assured me that things would go well and she would be certain to talk with Kelly after the surgery was complete. As she was walking away from the stretcher, I gave my permission to also talk to any of my friends who were with Kelly in the waiting room.

"They *all* know everything that's going on with me", I added.

The anesthetist walked in after Dr. Willard left and injected my IV with the anesthetic, Versed. I played the "counting backwards" game in my head...100, 99, 98, 97...

The next thing I knew, it was 9:45pm—my surgery finished—and I was awakening in a private room. Through foggy eyes, my conscious state returning, I began to recognize that Kelly and Michelle, along with Marge and her husband, Ed were all standing at the foot of my bed. Feeling intoxicated, but deliriously happy—both from the drugs and the fact that the surgery was over—I initiated a chatty conversation that was apparently entertaining to all of them. One-liners were coming out of me as if I were onstage at a Comedy Club!!!

After about an hour of this, they decided I was a little too loopy and should get some rest.

As my daughter and her friend were kissing me good-bye, I asked Marge if she brought her pillow since she was "scheduled" to spend the two nights with me in the hospital. Apologetically, Marge said, "I think I am coming down with something, my throat is scratchy and I think its best if I don't stay tonight. I don't want to give you anything."

Although I was disappointed, I said, "You're right. I don't want to take a chance that I may get sick with the flu while I am trying to recover from this surgery."

"I'll call tomorrow", she said as Ed waved good-bye and they left my room. I remember thinking, "*Hmmm...the best laid plans...*"

Before Kelly and Michelle left, Kelly set up my CD to play meditative music and then placed the headset over my ears. As I was relaxing, she covered my eyes with a black satin sleep mask that had "Do Not Disturb" sewn onto it—a thoughtful gift from Diana.

"Kelly, will you please hand me the PCA[3] pump button before you leave?" I asked, as they were starting out the door.

Taking advantage of the handy device, I pressed the button to administer some pain medicine and it wasn't long before I drifted off to sleep.

As in any hospital, the nurses and their assistants came in and out of the room throughout the night, taking temperatures, blood pressures, checking IVs, dressings and drains. Each time they woke me, I had them rewind my CD player and after they left, I pressed the Start button.

At 7:00 am the next morning, I was startled awake by a cheerful nurse aide, who wanted to check my vital signs and sit me up in a chair. Needless to say, I felt like I had been on an all night drunk.

After she finished taking my temperature and blood pressure, the aide leaned toward me, wrapped her arms around my shoulders and said she was going get me up and out of bed. I wasn't sure that this was such a good plan.

I slurred in a pleasant, but somewhat sarcastic tone: "Look, I am almost 5'11" and you are what...4'8"?

"5.0" even," she corrected me.

"No way" I said emphatically. "If you are helping me up and I start to go down...I want another person on the other side of me to help catch me."

The nurse aide promptly went in search of a second pair of arms.

Even in my drugged stupor, I was trying to think ahead and control the situation, knowing that if I fainted or started falling, I didn't want anyone grabbing my chest area, where drainage tubes and dressings were in abundance. So, I was not getting out of that bed until a second person was called in.

In the middle of this exchange, Dr. Willard came in. She examined me, checking under the dressings and had a look of satisfaction on her face. "I do good work", she bragged.

"I know you do", I concurred.

She asked if there was anything I needed. I just chuckled.

I proceeded to tell her that the nurses had complimented her throughout the night, saying that "Dr. W. thinks of everything when she writes her post-operative orders"...a couple of pain medications (in the event that one didn't work, the nurses already had an order for something different), anti-nausea medications, medications to start my bowels moving and sleep medicine. Dr. Willard smiled knowingly.

Still feeling woozy, I said, "The only thing I want is for you to discontinue this PCA pump. The medicine is making me feel like

I have a hangover and I don't like the feeling—I would rather concentrate on feeling strong, so I can get out of here as soon as possible."

"Done!" she said. "I have already written orders for pain medicine that you can take by mouth. If there is anything else you need, let the nurses know; otherwise, I will see you tomorrow."

Shortly after that, the nurse came in and removed the pump along with the I.V. Then she and the aide carefully assisted me to a chair, where they put a breakfast tray in front of me.

"Yum-m-my!!!" I growled sarcastically. Chicken broth, cherry jell-o and apple juice. Even on a good day, those "clear liquids" would not appeal to me.

Pushing the tray aside, I drank some water and prayed that Sharon—who would be visiting me at lunch—would bring the Steak 'n Shake milkshake that she promised.

Later that morning, I got a phone call from Trish, who had been "scheduled" to pick me up and drive me home the next morning, following my discharge.

"How are you feeling?" Trish asked tentatively.

"Not too bad," I replied. "I can't wait to go home to my own bed."

I know," she said sympathetically...and then she started to cough uncontrollably. "I just wanted to let you know that I won't be able to pick you up tomorrow. I have the flu and I don't want you to get it. Maybe Marge can pick you up?"

"No...Marge also has the flu," I said.

"Well, do you think you can find someone else? If not, I will be happy to come and get you," she graciously offered.

"No thanks," I said. "I really don't want to be exposed to the flu at this point." *Two down.* I was getting a little nervous.

At lunchtime, another tray was delivered. This time it included a creamy soup, milk and some pudding. Obviously, I had progressed to full liquids. *Why do things look so unappealing on a hospital food tray?* I pushed it away as Sharon walked in with a Steak and Shake bag in her hand. *Yahoo!!! Sharon saved the day!!!* As we visited, I slowly sipped the vanilla milkshake, savoring each mouthful.

Following Sharon's "shift", Sue was scheduled to sit with me for a few hours. On time as always, Sue arrived and I began telling her about the surgery.

The phone rang and Sue picked it up. As she handed me the phone, she said "It's Priscilla".

Priscilla is a nurse friend of mine from San Diego, who was scheduled to fly into Orlando the next day. We had planned her visit so that she could care for me during my first three days at home, since Kelly was away at a horse show.

As I hung up the phone, I shook my head and said: "I can't believe this! Everyone that I had scheduled to help me after surgery has the flu!"

I thought I had planned so carefully...now I didn't know what I was going to do.

"Don't worry," Sue said. "I'll work with Marge and put together a schedule. You just concentrate on getting well and let us take care of this."

Sue stayed with me until late that evening. She offered to spend the night and then drive me home in the morning. I knew that her husband had just flown back to town after being gone for a few weeks.

I was getting very drowsy. "Why don't you go home and spend some time with John", I suggested, "and then you can come back in the morning and take me home. I'll be okay tonight." Reluctantly, Sue conceded, and began to gather her things.

As she was going out the door, she said, "Marge and I are working on your home care. Kay will stay with you after I drop you off tomorrow and Jo has offered to spend the night." Apparently she had been working the phones, while I napped during her visit. "You are a good friend", I said sleepily.

As I was drifting off to sleep, there was a knock at my door. Peeking into the room, Kay, a pediatric nurse practitioner, was grinning from ear to ear.

"What in the world are you doing here this late?" I asked.

"I wanted to get out of the house for a little while, so I thought I would visit," she laughed. "I flashed my hospital badge at the nurses, so they didn't have a problem with me coming in!"

"*No kidding?!!* I understand that you are taking care of me tomorrow afternoon?"

"Yes and I wanted to do an assessment before we got you home," she joked, but in a very solemn manner.

"You're a crazy person!" I chuckled.

After visiting about fifteen minutes, Kay saw that I was falling asleep while she was talking. So she said her goodbyes and told me she would see me the next day.

I soon learned that the second post-operative night was not going to be as peaceful as the first. Without the PCA pump, I was awakened more easily.

Although, I wasn't alert the night before when they wheeled me to my room, I assumed I was *very* close to the nurse's station. I was absolutely correct. All night long, I heard the nurses talking; doors slamming; and was startled awake each time someone came into my room (which was at least every hour!!!)

Because I had taken pain medicine before I went to sleep, I refused the sleeping pill that they had offered earlier in the evening. I didn't want to feel the after effects in the morning. *That was a big mistake!!!*

Noticing that I wasn't sleeping, the nurses continued to ask through the night if I wanted the sleeping pill. "No thanks." I said. My plan was to be alert and ready to leave as soon as Dr. Willard wrote the discharge order.

By 7:30am the next morning, with the help of a taller nurse aide, I was up in a chair, dressed and waiting to go home. The day-shift nurse walked in, did a double take and said: "You don't have a discharge order."

"Don't worry," I said confidently. "I will get one."

About an hour later, Dr. Willard walked in and laughed. "The nurses *said* you wanted to go home, but I didn't think you would be ready to walk out the door!!"

"Oh yeah...I am MORE than ready. I *cannot* stay in that bed for one more night. What they say is true...you can't get any rest in the hospital!"

After looking at the dressings and listening to my lungs, Dr. Willard gave me the thumbs up. "Was Dr. Rotatori here yet?"

"Yes, he was here at 7:00am. He said I looked good and gave me an appointment next week to remove the drains."

"O.K.", she said. "You're out of here. I will see you in my office in two weeks."

I gathered my things and tried to eat a little from the breakfast tray but the only thing I could get down was the yogurt.

A short time later, Sue arrived to take me home. She received the discharge instructions from the nurse as the aide assisted me into the wheelchair. Two days post-mastectomy, I was feeling pretty good.

I was on my way home...and on my way to recovery.

6. Starting the Recovery

For it is in the giving that we receive—St. Francis of Assisi

As I have said over and over, it is good to have friends. And I have some very loyal and generous friends. Little did I know that every day in the coming year, I would be thanking one of them for some gesture that offered their love and support.

Lorraine's words kept echoing in my mind: "When your friends want to do something for you...let them. This is a time to learn to receive and allow your loved ones to give."

On the way home from the hospital, Sue explained that until Kelly was able to come home, she and Marge had scheduled some of my nurse friends to care for me.

Once again, I realized that Divine Intervention had taken place. The friends that I had originally scheduled for this "job" were not nurses and, although they would have been eager to take good care of me, I doubt they would have been able to cope with the dressings and drainage—that were part of the post-operative care—without gagging. Instead, I would have friends who, even though some were not currently working as nurses, would not hesitate to "milk" my drains and measure the drainage; change my dressings, and look carefully at my suture lines for any signs of infection.

When Sue and I arrived at my house, Kay was waiting patiently in my driveway. Both she and Sue escorted me inside. Once I was settled, Sue proceeded to review with Kay the instructions that had been outlined by the nurse on discharge. Kay looked through my "hospital goodie bag" and began unpacking. She pulled out sterile gauze dressings, tape, measuring cups for drainage, and the plastic breathing apparatus that would help my lungs to stay clear. As Kay thrust the apparatus into my hands, she started to morph into Nurse Ratchet before my very eyes!

"Here, you need to do this", she ordered. "Every hour!"

Rolling my eyes, I placed the mouthpiece between my lips and started to inhale. As I watched the first two balls rise with my inhalation, Kay shouted: "Breathe deeper!"

I breathed more deeply and the third ball rose up into the plastic tube. "Good job!" Kay said approvingly. I looked at the clock and thought, *"Oh Lord...It's going to be a long day."*

Sue smiled as she wished me luck with my new caregiver—the person who used to be my friend, Kay. After Sue left, Kay escorted me to my bedroom and helped me to lie down while she began to prepare lunch.

Every hour—on the dot—Nurse Ratchet came into my bedroom with the breathing apparatus. Needless to say, I had no problems with post-operative pneumonia!

Before I took a nap, I asked Kay if she would send an email out to my family and friends to let them know that the surgery was over. She was happy to oblige:

> Sent: Friday, December 12, 2003 8:08 PM
> To: My Prayer Group
> Subject: Metamorphosis-Part III
> Hello from Carla via her nurse! She wanted everyone to know that she is blessed that surgery went extremely well and she is now at home. Yes, her muscles are sore but she is a real trouper—walking, moving her arms and getting around quite well. She needs to keep her strength by resting often, as she tires easily.
> She will talk to everyone in a few days when she feels better. She thanks all of you for your prayers and positive thoughts. Keep them coming!!
> Love, Carla via Kay

I could hear the cheers in my head as I read the responses that came back...

> Hooray!
> Talked to your mom last night and already had the update. Feels like a brick wall hit your chest, huh? Well, you can't go anywhere but up from there. At least you are in your own bed. I have been continuously thinking about you and offering prayers and rosaries.
> Will wait for the OK to call, but will leave that up to you to signal.
> Love, Maur
>
> Hi Kay—Thanks for taking such good care of Carla. We appreciate it. Tell Carla I am thinking about her and keeping her in my prayers.
> Love, Linda

Hi Carla,

I am so glad that you are home and doing so well...didn't expect anything other!!! Hope you have a speedy recovery! Of course, we will miss you at Marge's tonight. My prayers continue. Take care. Olga

Carla,

I am thinking of you and wishing you were going with us tonight but know you need to rest. I am going to try and be there on Sunday. Do you need me to pick up some groceries? Any special requests? Has Kelly returned from her horse show yet? Call me. Diana

At about 9:30pm, the "nursing" staff changed shifts. Out with Kay and in with Jo, who would spend the night. When Jo arrived, I was awake and sitting up—ready for the sleepover! Jo approached to give me a hug—which I refused.

"You look great!" She said with amazement. "If you hadn't refused my hug, I would never know that you had surgery".

It was true.

Considering the fact that it was only my second day post-op, I felt surprisingly good. I had virtually no pain, but was not looking forward to my first night at home. Due to the drains on both sides of my chest, I would have to sleep on my back; and since I am a side sleeper, I knew that I would have some trouble with back soreness.

Jo and I talked for about an hour before we decided to call it a night. Jo wanted to sleep on the couch to be closer to my room in the event that I needed her. However, I insisted that she sleep in the upstairs guest room.

"I have this bell," I said. "If I need anything, I will ring it and you can come down". We tested the bell to be sure that she could hear it upstairs. Although she didn't think either of us would sleep soundly, Jo set the clock to be sure that she would awaken in time to administer my antibiotics.

Even though I preferred my own bed to the one in the hospital, there was a definite advantage to being able to raise the head and knees on the electric hospital bed, thus keeping pressure off my back.

At 1:30 am, my back was hurting, and since I couldn't raise myself up off the bed, I began to ring the bell for Jo. She came downstairs immediately, and helped me sit up...and then stand so that I could stretch my back. After stretching for a few minutes, Jo helped me back into bed and eased me to a lying position. She then set up my meditation CD, helped me with the headset and within a short time, I was back to sleep.

At 5:30am, I became restless again; sleeping in one position was not easy for me. Even before I had a chance to ring the bell, I looked over and Jo was standing at my doorway ready to assist. She scared the heck out of me!!!

Apparently, it was time for my antibiotic and the alarm had wakened her. Once again we started the routine—I got up and stretched, took my pill, Jo helped me back to bed and I fell asleep until 7:30am, when I called for help to get up.

Jo and I lounged around for breakfast and half the morning, before we decided that it was time for my first post-op shower and dressing change.

Unable to lift my arms, it was quite a feat for Jo to shampoo and rinse my hair—while I was in the shower and she stood outside of the tub. There was water everywhere! Jo was soaking wet as she cleaned the puddles of water from the floor, joking that it might have worked better if she had gone in the shower with me!

When it came time to dry and style my hair, it was obvious that Jo had no experience in that department. She tried and tried, but could not make it look at all close to my own style. And, of course, I could be of no help.

"Just give me a bag!" I suggested. She laughed at me.

"Thank goodness, I don't have to show myself in public." I said while looking in the mirror at the disaster that she created. We giggled hysterically like two school girls.

As lunchtime was approaching, Jo called her husband to ask him to pick up some salads from our favorite Greek café. What Jo didn't realize though, was that she called the wrong restaurant to put in the order. So, when Craig arrived an hour or so later with lunch, we all realized the mistake. Luckily, Craig is a patient and forgiving husband.

Having enjoyed lunch, we chatted for awhile when the doorbell rang. Jo got up to answer it and there stood Sharon.

"Hi y'all!" She greeted us with her southern twang. "Nurse Sharon reporting for duty!"

As I thanked Craig for lunch, Jo gathered her things and reviewed the morning activities with Sharon, along with the medication schedule.

"Okay Sharon, I will leave the patient in your competent hands!" Jo said, as she and Craig went out the door.

As I said goodbye, I sent up a prayer thanking God for the special friends with whom I have been so blessed.

That evening, my daughter came over. Just returning from a three day horse show, she had two days off and would spend them caring for her mom. In 27 years, it was the first time that our roles were reversed and Kelly really had the opportunity to be my caregiver. It was a role that she accomplished with patience, humor and love. After those two days, I knew that, when the time came, she would be a wonderful mother!

Four days after surgery, I was able to get to my computer to send out my own update of the recent surgery and post-op activities.

Sent: Friday, December 14, 2003 7:25 PM
To: My Prayer Group
Subject: Metamorphosis-Part III-4th Post op day
"Treasure every moment that you have! And treasure it more because you shared it with someone special...special enough to have some of your time!"—Benjamin Franklin

My...my...my...how time flies...especially when you are on drugs!!!

Well—mission completed—and I am back in the co-pilot's seat (whoever wrote "GOD is my co-pilot" is dead wrong—God is THE PILOT which has been proven to me over and over in these past few weeks).

Relevant to that is when I only had about a day and a half to prepare for my hospitalization. I worked frantically to set up a "project management plan" (as Janis called it), developing an EXCEL spreadsheet with everyone's home phone numbers, cell phone and work numbers and in my "comments column" I had a "schedule" of those who agreed to stay with me during the hospitalization, discharge and through the weekend, so that each caregiver would know who was on the next "shift"—so to speak. As it happened, *everyone* that I had scheduled to stay with me—either during the night at the hospital, taking me home from the hospital or caring for me at night at home—ended up with the dreaded flu.

However, Marge (who was sick) and Sue (who was not) worked out a schedule...and by the time I was ready to leave the hospital, they had "the perfect plan" worked out, which included all of my "old hospital buddies", who were willing and able to care for me. I couldn't have asked for better nursing care than I received from them!

So, my appreciation to everyone who had anything to do with my very easy transition from hospital to home—including Marge and Sue for coordinating this effort.

Also, thanks to Gay for staying with Kelly during the surgery. Thank you to Sue, who after spending 8 hours with me in the hospital on Thursday, came back on Friday morning to take me home.

...to Sharon for the delicious Steak and Shake milkshake that you brought for Thursday's lunch and for the food you brought on Saturday. To Kay aka Nurse Ratchett (just kidding), who MADE me do my inspirator EVERY hour after I got home—as the doctor ordered! (Also thanks for the late night visit on Thursday—guess it pays to be a honcho at Florida Hospital.)

...and to Jo, who graciously spent the night on Friday and who helped me with my shower and washed my hair on Saturday (amongst other nursely duties). Jo...keep your day job, since we know that you are not—and will never be—a hair stylist (although you did better than Kelly, who made me look like Rod Stewart!!) Thanks to Jo's husband, Craig, for bringing lunch from Athen's Cafe—even though Jo called the order into Athena's (the wrong restaurant!!).

Thanks to Kelly, who has experienced her first inkling of what it's going to be like taking care of me in my old age. Her omelet's are delicious, her nursing skills with the dressing changes are up to par with some of my cronies, but I have to admit, her hairstyling skills will only work if and when I become a rock star!!

Also, thanks to Jacqueline, who I haven't seen for 8 years, for getting up early this morning to make me homemade bread and chicken soup and for bringing her beautiful family over to deliver it before church this evening.

And...to all of you, who have felt "horrible" or "guilty" (or whatever crazy feelings that you have expressed) because you couldn't be with me due to illness or distance or other commitments...I thank you the most, because I know that feeling...but want you to know that your thoughts and prayers and your phone calls and emails expressing encouragement have been just as important as being with me.

I am blessed to have *all of you* in my life; and because of you, things have actually seemed quite easy, believe it or not.

Tomorrow, I should hear the news about the pathology of the lymph nodes...so again I ask you to keep me in your prayers.

I didn't think I would be in the Christmas spirit this year, but I am beginning to understand its true meaning. It's not about the lights and the presents, it's about love...and I want you to know that I am constantly feeling the love from all of you and don't want you to go one day without knowing how much I love you all.

I am in the healing light...

Carla

My dear Car:

So good to know that you are back at the keyboard and have not lost any of your eloquent style. Just wish someone had a digital camera so I could see some of those hairstyles.

Dave is being my mail-boy tomorrow so I can get a package off to you, something for the body and something for the spirit. Plus you will get a new supply of Lourdes' water direct ship AND with an order form so you can get refills for yourself...or others when you have moved on from this time.

I do know that guilty feeling about not being able to be one of the lucky ones, who can cook, clean, bathe, torture and harass you directly. And although you absolve us, it does not make us feel much better. But I am planning on a trip at the end of Jan or early Feb. I am waiting to see what your treatment plan will be.

How bad does it hurt, by the way? Are the drains still in? You are in my daily prayers and thoughts, and will continue to be

Love Maur

Carla~

"Trooper" is an understatement! You are utterly amazing—but you already know that. It's good to hear that you're back home and able to recoup in your own environs. You'll be back at the gym in no time at all! But for now, just take it slow please.

I am so bummed that the flu descended upon me this week. I really wanted to be there to be your nurse. Although you are probably better off that Nurse Ratchet, Jr. had to stay home! Sending my love and wishes for a speedy and uneventful recovery.

~Priscilla

Six days after surgery, it was D-DAY! (That is, **D**rain removal **D**ay.) After days of "milking" the tubes, draining and measuring the fluid, I was anxious—no, actually excited—to take this next step in my healing process. However, only *after* the tubes were removed, did I realize how bothersome—not painful—they really were hanging from my chest like two extra appendages!

Date: 12/16/03
To: My Prayer Group
Subject: 6th Post-Op Day
'Peace is the state where love abides and seeks to share itself.'
—Gandhi

Hello all!

I just got back from the plastic surgeon's office...my great friend Sue was kind enough to drive me back and forth. While in the waiting room, another serendipitous event—I met Diane (another breast cancer patient that I had only spoken with on the phone a few weeks ago—referred to me by a trainer at the gym). She was there for a pre-op visit—as she is having her final surgery tomorrow morning.

Anticipating a little pain from the removal of my drains, I had taken a Percocet prior to arriving at the office and was a little spacey, but listened closely as Diane started giving me a "blow-by-blow" of her experience. She had me VERY nervous about having my drains removed, because she said: "Get ready—having the drains removed was the worst pain" of every thing she had been through!!! In fact, she could only tolerate having one removed and waited to have the second one removed during her second surgery. YIKES!!!!

Just as I was about to get on board the Panic Train, Sue (God bless her) reminded me of my high tolerance for pain and had me demonstrating deep breathing techniques. As soon as they called me to the back, I started asking about the "pain" and was assured that it was "similar to stubbing your toe—a little burn and then it would go away". They told me it was OK to SCREAM (Oh...that's comforting?!?!?!)

Remembering Lorraine's advice (from my last plastic surgeon visit), I asked Dr. Rotatori if I could have *both* drains taken out *at the same time*, a request which was accommodated.

So, I got up on the table with a nurse on each side of me and was told to hold onto the sides of the table.

I said: "Wait...*you* hold on—I need to say a little prayer—and Sue needs to hold my feet for her healing touch".

Then, they told me to take a deep breath and on the count of three, they yanked them out!!! I swear I felt a *small* tug—and was expecting the worst to start—but they were out and the dressings were already on! I must have had an out of body experience, because it did not hurt at all!!!

You cannot imagine how happy I was to have those "appendages" removed. Although the nurses said I might regret losing my "two balls"! Of course, instead of four—now I only had two remaining (that's a joke, mom...it means I have "balls"—get it???)

Dr. Rotatori and I discussed the very real possibility of having my eyes and a mini face-lift done in a few months when he inserts my implants. He thought it would not be a problem and said that they even give discounts on elective procedures which are done at the same time as an insurance-approved procedure. So, start sending your contributions today!!!

I left the office feeling WONDERFUL...free of the hanging drains, with an "I am a GREAT PATIENT" sticker on my chest (an alternative to the variety of lollipops that the nurses offered me--they had NO sugar free, can you believe it)!!!

Sue asked if I needed to run any errands on the way home, so we stopped at Dillard's and bought a couple of new "soft" bras—size 36C (ALREADY a size bigger than I was—uh huh!!) Only after I got into the changing room and took off my sweater did I realize that I had worn my "GREAT PATIENT" sticker all through Dillard's. Sue said she thought I wanted everyone to know how well I did. OMG! Thanks, Sue.

Anyway, ANOTHER great day in my Metamorphosis.

OH, Sorry, I guess you were wondering about the pathology report—I called the doc's office when I got home. They haven't received a report yet, so I will let you all know when I hear something.

Til then...I will sign off and get ready for my date...as we are going to Trish's Open House for a couple of hours (with my new, sexy bra! —Don't worry, dad, he won't see it)
Carla

Hey Carla~

I remember my drains burning a bit when they were removed after the lumpectomy and tummy tuck; as well as face lift (wow, I've had a lot of surgery), but it was nothing in light of what I had already been through. Glad you are out and about and partying a little bit.

When will you be allowed to drive a car?

See you tomorrow night around 6 p.m. Sandi and I may join you for dinner if you are up to company. If you are not, just say the word, as we don't want you to feel you have to entertain us.

We'll be stopping at Publix. Let me know if there is anything I can pick up for you, milk, bread, M&M's?
Barbara

> Barb~
>
> Doc said I could drive when I can open and close the door and maneuver the steering wheel (turning around to check behind me, etc.) I am looking forward to seeing you and Sandi tomorrow. Marge may join us, as well. Yes...let's have an M&M appetizer, then some chocolate soup as the main dish and a chocolate torte for dessert.
> Carla

Car~

What a riot. This is like reading a novel, but non-fiction.

I am a firm believer in prayer too, but I think the drain removal experience has something to do with your high pain tolerance. It should please you to know that I am considering a change of jobs this year if I can find something that I WANT to do. I applied for a case manager and clinical trials coordinator at the Joyce Murtha Breast Cancer Center in Windber, even before I knew about your diagnosis.

Like you say, what will be, will be, but I really would like to look into the opportunity, especially after this has happened to you.

In closing, Dillard's is one of my favorite stores in the whole US. So you have not lost your sense of good taste (except for the patient sticker on your chest).

Love Maur

P.S. Get the eyes done, but why a mini facelift? That takes expression out of the face and makes you look like Michael Jackson. Even Nichole Kidman has done something that has taken the softness out of her face and now she is looking mask-like. She should have called me first for advice...

Carla:

Your healing process continues to be an inspiration to me. I can identify with the "removing of the drains" scenario. After my breast reduction surgery, of course I had those damn drains hanging from me like an additional set of teats—though unlike you, I didn't take the Percocet (I'm such a control freak)...no buffer for me. The darn stinking nurse yanked those puppies out....I almost kicked her with my TIMBERLAND boots—it hurt like hell, but I survived (strong woman).

I am glad to hear that you are getting out and about. Be careful with that "elective surgery"...don't want you to get hooked and become like the $1MILLION dollar Barbie-woman. Lynne

Carla,
Your experiences are truly evidence in my mind that the Lord works in mysterious ways...always looking for us to just believe and have faith. Well, He has my attention!!!

I am so glad that everything is going so well for you....Know that you are thought of and prayed for each day.

Merry Christmas and here's to a brand new year of wonderful, fulfilling experiences. Olga

Carla, your emails are heartwarming, hilarious, and deeply touching—a beautiful role model for all of us. Have saved each email to put into my "Carla Folder"—for us to reminisce together...at the river, your home, the streets of NY, or wherever—for years to come. Much Love, Pat S.

Carla—A.K.A. "Great Patient"...
You are a "piece of work"...mighty fine work! Your attitude continues to inspire me! Have FUN tonight and take good care. Love you, Sue

Date: 12/17/03
To: My Prayer Group
Subject: 7th Day Post-op
'What matters most is how well you walk through the fire.'
—Charles Bukowski

You won't believe this—I stubbed my toe this morning...wasn't watching where I was going and BAM right into the foot of my lounge chair. Damn, it hurt...but only for a few seconds. (Much worse than having the drains removed!)

Well, I have some good news!!!! Dr. Willard just called and said: "Guess who doesn't have cancer in ANY of her lymph nodes?"

Holding my breath, I asked: "Who??" and she said: "YOU!!!!" Whoooooopppppppeeeeeeeeeeeeeeeeeee! I have an appointment with the Oncologist on December 31st to determine the treatment phase of this ordeal.

Thank God. Again, I have been blessed and can attribute it to ALL of your prayers, novenas, masses and prayer chains. Thank you, thank you, thank you!

The bad news for my family is that—after much consideration—I have decided not to fly to North Carolina for our "Very Baldo Christmas 2003-A Return to the Outer Banks". I am not sure who is going to sing "Sisters" with JanJan (from the movie White Christmas with Rosemary Clooney and Vera Allen), since that has been our tradition for years. (Damn...and this year, I know the words!).

Anyway, I have been assured that my father is placing a picture of Kelly and me on the dining table, so that the family can talk about us and reminisce about all the trouble we caused during previous reunions. I will miss being there.

The good news is that I called Delta and they are giving me a credit on both tickets to be used within the year without a change fee.

So, it looks like I will be banging on a few friends' doors this Christmas for a "hand-out"...but, perhaps Kelly and I can rehearse the song and dance "Sisters" for the next week, so that we can "pay" for our dinner with some excellent entertainment!

Again...thank you all for your support and prayers. Thank you for the flowers, the lunches, the dinners, the buttermilk, the phone calls and the visits. And I forgot to acknowledge Michelle, Kelly's best friend and my second daughter, for her ability to keep a secret (something Kelly said she could never do) during the crazy time when I was scrambling during my preparation for the unscheduled hospitalization. Michelle "pulled off" a surprise birthday party for Kelly last Thursday...a birthday that Kelly said "was the best one in her life"...boy, she ain't kidding, huh?

I know that I have regained the true perspective about what Christmas REALLY is and I believe that it will be a joyful time for all of us. Love and blessings to all for a Happy Holiday season!!!!

Carla

P.S. I forgot to extend my appreciation to Judy, my hairdresser, who spent half of her day off on Monday to come to my house to cut my hair (Kelly conned her into cutting hers also) and to Sue and Jo, who were so generous with their time by driving me to my doctors' appointments.

Also, I wanted you to know that my whole family extends their appreciation to all of my local friends who were "there for me" when they couldn't physically be here (actually, because I had so much local support, I didn't want them to fly/drive down on such short notice). They are sending prayers to bless each and every one of you.

Carla,
What wonderful news! I love getting your e-mails. You are so positive about life. You are an inspiration. I'll call you for movie and dinner after my folks and sister (with her 3 kids) leave after Christmas. I get sad when my folks leave so I will need a good laugh from you!!
Love, Kay

Thanks Carla...
Hope you are having a good day with no pain. I hope the sun is out and you can feel it on your face...its overcast and ugly (winter is upon us) here in beautiful downtown DC.
I spoke with Jerry this morning. He asked about you and I was happy to give him the great news that you are cancer free...he replied that "our prayers have been answered."
I'm gonna scoot...although I will miss you at the "2003: Back to the Outer Banks-Family Reunion" (and no we won't talk about you—not badly anyway).
You're making the right choice to stay put...just heal and be well, sister friend. By the way, what's up with the job? Last I heard it was looking good. AND I understand there is a man in your life. God, you are ending 2003 on a high note...
Take care, say hi to Kelly Jelly Belly for me.
Hugs and Kisses,
Cookie

Carla,
Can't tell you how elated we are to hear your GREAT NEWS. Praise the Lord! Of course, we will continue to pray for you through the days to come.
After I pulled up your e-mail, I called Jacqueline on her cell to see if she had heard. Their computer had crashed & I have NO idea what she meant when she was telling me how it happened. Anyway, I barely got out the words & then it happened. You might have heard our screams of happiness from your place!!!
Big hugs from both of us!
Love, Judy

Carolyn~
WHAT an answer to our prayers!!! You made my day! I am smiling through glistening eyes!!!
Love,
Sharolyn

Hey Mimi:
Just got home from a Holiday Dinner with my "supper club." It's 10:24 PM. Great news from Dr. Willard!!! Our prayers are answered! I am bummed that you won't be at the Outer Banks reunion, but it makes sense. Heal completely and be ready for the next steps.
I love you.
Jan Jan

Carla,
GREAT NEWS!! What absolutely FANTASTIC NEWS!!
Trish

Carla,
Oh, all our prayers have been answered!! What a glorious day this is! Hooray—and God be praised again by those of us who should praise Him more often.

I am sorry that you will not be with your family, but surely the good news outweighs the disappointment.

So does this mean you do not need to have second line treatment of any kind? If not, I will proceed to begin my travel plans but do not want to make any arrangements until I have a go ahead from you.

You are so right about the true meaning of Christmas. I will add my special thanks for you this year as we sing our Christmas Eve liturgy. Dave and I both sing with our contemporary choir, as music is so much a part of who I am—going back to the "Annie Get Your Gun Days" in the high school play.
Love and Joy, Maur

Although I talked about having chemotherapy, I didn't really feel that I was going to need it. With the belief that I was coming to the end of my journey with cancer, I assumed that my emails would soon be coming to a halt. I wrote—what I thought would be—one of my last.

Date 12/18/03
To: My Prayer Group
Subject: 8th Post-op day
'May we live in peace without weeping. May our joy outline the lives we touch without ceasing. And may our love fill the world, angel wings tenderly beating.' —An Irish Blessing

Well gang...

You must be tired of all of these emails, so this will be the last for a little while...at least until I see the oncologist on December 31st. At that point, we may move to Metamorphosis Part IV-Treatment—but I hope not. (Part I-Diagnosis; Part II-Surgery; Part III-Post-op)

Once again, Jo Manion came to the rescue today and picked me up at noon to drive me to see Dr. Willard at 2:15pm. We stopped for lunch at TGIFridays and shared a pecan-crusted chicken salad—my favorite—which was FABULOUS!

After we arrived in the doctor's office, we started to chat with another woman who had a bilateral mastectomy named Marlene. She couldn't believe that I had just had surgery last Wednesday. (I had on my leather pants and boots and a red sweater—cause it's COLD here—in the 50's) and I was lookin' FINE (right, Jo?).

It's amazing how quickly you get into conversations when you share the same diagnosis. Marlene had her surgery in May and her implants placed in November and she was saying how tired she was. She was astounded that I had only stayed in the hospital for 2 days—(she stayed in 4 days)—and that I was feeling so good only a week after surgery.

I told her about the Healing CD that I listened to for three weeks prior to surgery and we began talking about the research regarding guided imagery and affirmations. Jo suggested that Marlene might benefit from a CD called "Healing Trauma." She gave her the name of the website, where she could order the CD. Actually, some of you may want to check out this site www.healthjourneys.com . Go onto the site and scroll to Audio Spa, then try the sample "Spa Treatment" to hear Belleruth Naparstek's voice and a guided imagery. There are tapes for Stress, Pain, Relationship (I gotta get THAT one), Depression, Headache, Smoking, etc.

Anyway, Marlene felt that she "was guided to meet us today" to help her overcome the trauma that she experienced during her surgery. Things like this have been happening to me more than you know—since the day I was told that I had cancer. Perhaps, when one is "stopped in their tracks", one becomes more spiritually aware. The first thing I did was surrender to God and trust that whatever the process and the outcome—it would be what is best for me and will put me on the Path that I am to be in this life.

Divine Intervention is a powerful thing and it happens to all of us on a daily basis. My wish for all of you is not to have to experience any type of life-threatening illness, but to benefit from my experience. Evaluate your everyday life and make sure that you are taking the time in your day to recognize that Intervention and to give Thanks. Also, know that "things are as they should be"...which is what I continue to believe.

One last thing, Dr. Willard said that because of the aggressive type of cancer cells that they found, most likely I will have to have chemo. So, yes, I guess one of my Christmas gifts to myself will be a wig or two...I just have to decide if I want to go blonde, red or brunette. Whoever wants to accompany me on that shopping trip is welcome. As you can imagine, it will be a party!!!!

Lots of Love,
Carla aka Mimi van Breastus

Dear Carla,

My computer has been down for a couple of days but I think it is back up and running now! Congratulations on the very good news regarding the pathology reports! Praise God!

Judy and I were talking about how much we miss you and how much we wish you had become our sister-in-law. But you will always have a big, special place in our hearts. We will always be there for you, too. I have always respected you and loved your attitude on life, but now I am truly inspired by it.

If there is anything I can help you with, I would love to be able to do that. It would be great to be able to see you again, too. I hope you and Kelly have a very special Christmas here; I know how badly you wanted to go to North Carolina. You will be in our prayers.

Love, Jacqueline

Carla: I've been thinking about you all week but have not been on email. I started vacation on Monday and could not bear to bring myself to the computer. Now I'm regretting it, but thrilled to get all your messages at once and thrilled with the news. My mouth watered when you mentioned Athena's and I too love the pecan crusted chicken salad (minus the mandarin oranges) at Friday's! I will call you this weekend as it sounds like you are rebounding well and available to talk.

I am off until the 5th so please let me know what I can do to help. If you'd like, I'd be happy to come over on the 31st and escort you to your appointment with the Oncologist. I might be able to translate for you!

Love, Wendy

Carla~
GREAT NEWS!!!!
Love, Your Bro

Carla...

Once again, I am inspired and so appreciate the deep level of sharing through your emails. I do hope you are taking Trish's suggestion and pulling this together for a book! It would be a fabulous journey to share with others...your insights are so right-on and such good reminders for all of us!

I had just popped your Christmas card in the mail when I read that you plan to stay home for the holiday. I imagine it was a difficult decision, but now you can just rest and recoup without the stress of travel (the airport scene leaves much to be desired since 9-11. I really gear myself up for an altered state each time I have to slip through the skies). Well, I, for one, look forward to your next email.
Take good care,
Love, Sue

Hey Carla-
What do you think about an impromptu get-together Saturday night with Olga, Brenda, me & whomever else—at either your house or mine? Count me in on shopping for the wigs; I'm sure it will be quite entertaining!
Love, Nadine

Carla:

Again I can identify with you...NASA offers the Desk Top Spa on our computers (maybe that's one of the reason's that NASA is the #1 place to work...ha ha) and I have listened to many of the treatments.

My "ah ha" moments have occurred twice in my life; the first, when the doctor treating Dad in Pittsburgh told me that there was a 2% chance of his surviving pancreatitis. It was at that moment that I surrendered and placed all of my burdens at Gods feet, and prayed for strength...the second time was when my marriage ended...and I believe that is when my second transformation came about. Today, I am more spiritually aware...I am happier than I have ever been and I believe I look better (nothing wrong with that!!!).

You're on the right path.
...I love you.
Ann

7. Beginning the "New" Year

'We judge ourselves by what we think we are capable of doing;
others judge us by what we have already done.'

—Henry Wadsworth Longfellow

Heading into the New Year, I was hopeful that my problems were behind me and the next year would prove less challenging than the previous one. At this point, my social calendar consisted of going to see the plastic surgeon every two weeks, so that the nurse could "inflate" my expanders. By injecting 100cc of saline into the temporary implants, this process helped stretch the skin over the breast area in order to prepare a "pocket" large enough to hold the permanent implants.

With that being the current 'highlight' of my life, I couldn't wait to get back to the gym.

Additionally, after 10 months of being unemployed, I was looking forward to starting the year with a new job and a refreshingly new attitude and with the desire to live each day to the fullest.

On the last day of the year—New Year's Eve day—I had, what I hoped was my last appointment with my oncologist.

> Date: Wed, 31 Dec 2003
> To: My Prayer Group
> Subject: Metamorphosis - Part IV
> Well, I hope your Christmas/Hannakuh/Kwanza was jolly...
> I am sitting here finishing up a glass of champagne, on this early eve of the New Year. My friend, Wendy, just left for her return to Tampa after having spent last evening and today with me. Wendy has alot of experience with breast cancer and worked for Aventis (the makers of Taxotere, a chemo drug for breast cancer), covering Moffett Cancer Center in Tampa. She generously took time out of her holiday vacation to come up to Orlando and accompany me to see the oncologist today.
> Of course, before we went to the oncologist, we strolled in and out of the shops on Park Avenue, and she is probably about $500 lighter than she was when she started!!!!
> Anyway, back to the champagne...I got to my appointment with Dr. Molthrop at 1:45pm, as scheduled—only to find out that he was ON VACATION!! So, Dr. Z., (one of his partners) came in and apologized for the screw-up and offered an

alternative—either make an appointment with Dr. Molthrop for next week...or he could see me today. So, I chose the latter.

Dr. Z. reviewed my pathology reports and came back into the room and said: "Your situation causes a little anxiety basically because (and these are all good things) 60% of your tumor was in situ (not extending beyond the area of origin), the tumor was only 1cm (very small), no cancer was noted in the lymph nodes (great news) BUT, the HER-2/neu (a genetic malfunction in the cells that caused the cancer) was positive (bad), but it was only 2+ (good). With these things in mind, and the fact that you had a bilateral mastectomy, your survival rate is 90% and chemotherapy would only give you another 1%."

He said that he wanted to run one more test, which would provide more explicit information about the HER-2/neu—called a FISH test, which will be a determining factor as to whether or not I should have chemo. So, that information will be available at my next appointment.

Needless to say, when we came out from the appointment, I was as confused as you probably are right now...but, Wendy was beaming, saying that we just heard some GREAT NEWS (huh?) and that we needed to celebrate before she left for Tampa.

Wendy seems to think that given all of the positives (as mentioned above) that the possibility of my having to start chemo may be only 25%—of course, all will be dependent upon the FISH test.

So, MORE prayers are requested that the FISH indicates my not needing chemo!!!

Other good news...I had myself inflated another 100cc yesterday—that went well. No pain, whatsoever...except for the **pained look** on Dr. Rotatori's face when I asked him "if (say this like Ahhhnold would say it) he was there to PUMP me up!!" Also, when I asked him how my breasts looked (healing, etc.) on a scale of 1-10, he said they were a 9+ !!!!! ...and the nurse told me that I don't need to wear a bra (OMG, the *last* time I heard those words was at age 13 when my mom said them!!!)

Lastly, and certainly not the least of this info—more good news...

I met with both the CFO and VP of Kelson Pharmacy on Monday. Following our conversation, they asked when I could start!! So, I am waiting for an offer letter and expect that in a week or so, I will be an employed member of the U.S. workforce once again. HALLELUIA!!!!

> Again, I want you to know that I can never thank all of you enough for your friendship, prayers and support over this past year. Here's to a joy-filled, healthy and abundant 2004 for all of us. HAPPY NEW YEAR!!!
> LOVE, Carla

Just before I hit the SEND button, I re-read my email and thought back to the earlier part of the day. I knew this email would create the same sensation that I had immediately after my visit with the oncologist. *Basically, my head was spinning!*

Recalling my post-appointment conversation with Wendy, I realized that I had placed my attention on all the positives that the doctor had discussed. Specifically, I focused on the number that Dr. Z. had mentioned when he talked about how chemotherapy would affect my survival rate—One per cent— **only 1 %**!!! My immediate reaction was: "I am NOT going to have chemotherapy for an additional survival rate of ONLY ONE PER CENT! Why should I withstand the nausea, vomiting, hair loss and weakness associated with having those chemicals put into my body for only one percent?!!"

I am NOT going to do it!!!

I hit the SEND button and the emails started to rush back to me.

> Carla:
> Great update, kiddo! And I'm so glad Wendy was with you. I'm totally concerned about why he said your case causes a little anxiety. Perhaps he was thinking you were not even considering chemo and wanted to do the test to determine whether you should?
> Also, do you think you'll get more saline pumped into your expanders, or are they big enough now? I'm so glad it didn't hurt. My neighbor would be shocked to hear that you had no pain, because she refused the reconstruction based on the experience of a friend who said that was the worst! Everything's relative, huh? Trish

> Hi Carla!!!
> Wow sounds great. I never needed the chemo stuff after my diagnosis and here I am 6 years down with a lot more living to do.
> I go under the knife myself on Monday. I am having a "waddle-ectomy"—yep a face lift. When you get to the ripe age

of almost 60, it is time for a little help. I'll have a perky face and you have your perky breasts.

Great news...hopefully the FISH test is negative.

Lynne

WOW Carla!

I am not sure if I truly understood everything... except the parts about champagne; bigger, painless new breasts and a new job, but I think that is enough for me to feel VERY happy for you. A big fat hug and a WHOOPEE!

As for me, I had a very good interview with the Joyce Murtha Breast Cancer Center Director of Nursing and existing RN case manager this past Monday. The position I am up for would be doing research (double blind) on HER2/neu and what effect the currently developed vaccine would have on preventing recurrence. Maybe you would meet criteria and would have to come here for the vaccine administration!

I think I did well, but like you, I am putting myself in God's hands, even if He does not mean for me to have this. Wish He would respond soon though, so that if it is not to be, I can accept and move on.

You are amazing to have so many good friends that can help with your education process. What a great resolution to everything, and all falling into place at the right time. Happy 2004—you deserve it!

Love and prayers

Maur

Hi Carla-

Thanks for the update. We will pray specifically for you not to need chemo. We wish you a healthier and Happy New Year! CONGRATULATIONS on the job! That's great news!

With Love,

Jacqueline, Jeff, Ashton & Tristan

Carla!!!

Praise the Lord!!!! Prayers are being answered!!!!! I have felt so guilty that I haven't gotten back to you since before Christmas... things have been so crazy around here.

Tonight at dinner I told Craig we had to call you to find out how the appointment went with the oncologist today...and then your e-mail arrived. I think you deserve to drink the whole bottle of champagne!!!

Hope you are relaxing...and enjoying the holiday...and YIKES! I guess you are going to be too busy for lunch now that you are a working woman again?

I am adding to the prayers....THAT THESE KELSON PEOPLE APPRECIATE YOU LIKE YOU DESERVE TO BE!!!!! I am so relieved for you...I probably have been more worried than you have been!!!!

Please take care... give yourself a hug for me! Oh yeah...you make me sick—not having to wear a bra!!!

Love ya, Jo

Carla,

What a wonderful letter. Hope the FISH test comes out neg. We do that test alot on our kids for their genetic workup. It's very thorough.

And starting a job!! Welcome back to the hectic pace of life.

Love, Kay

Carla/Mimi~

Fabulous news!!! I love you. JanJan

CARLA,

GREAT NEWS ALL AROUND. CONGRATULATIONS ON THE JOB AND REST ASSURED THAT THE PRAYERS WILL CONTINUE!!!!! LOVE, YOUR BRO AND SIS-IN-LAW

Carla,

We're so glad to hear the medical prognosis is looking so good. Congratulations on getting a new job! Hope to see you in Chicago sometime this year. Tom and Judy

Carla,

There is nothing nicer than to receive GOOD NEWS from you. It's about time. God has asked a lot from you the past year and I believe He will bless you in the future ones. Your strength and positive attitude merits mention. I can only hope that Kelly is paying attention. You are a wonderful example for her.

Thank you for keeping me posted and please know that you are always in my prayers. HAPPY NEW YEAR!

Love, Pat D.

Happy New Year, Carla! Thanks for the update...sounds very promising!! And you aren't going to be dropped from the prayer list any time soon!!! We all need prayer all the time....

> It was good to see you before Christmas. I am very jealous of the no bra thing......enjoy it!!! Olga

As I read my emails, I kept thinking about my visit with the oncologist. Even though the doctor—and Wendy sounded reassuring as to my future and the remote possibility that I would need chemotherapy...and even as the emails were coming back to me—congratulating me on the fact that I may not have to have chemo, I kept going back to the fact that I had been focused on the 1%, when both the doctor and Wendy focused on the 25%.

The emails arrived, one by one with their questions about the FISH test, and since I really did not grasp the concept of the HER-2/neu and how the FISH test would determine whether or not I should have chemo, I felt a need to further my own research into the unknown.

So, I logged onto Google and typed in the words: **HER-2/neu; FISH; Breast Cancer**. Several sites came up, so I started reading:

HER-2/neu, also referred to as HER-2 or cerB-2, is one of the more than 100,000 genes occurring in the nucleus of all human cells, including breast tissue cells. The HER-2 gene is a portion of genetic code that exists in everyone and plays a key role in the regulation of normal cell growth. The HER-2 gene helps cells grow, divide and repair themselves. Normally a person will have two copies of this gene for every cell. In approximately 25% to 30% of all breast cancer tumors, there are extra copies of this gene, which cause too many HER-2 proteins (receptors) to appear on the cell surface. This is referred to as HER-2 protein "over expression" or "amplification". These special proteins bind with other circulating growth factors to cause uncontrolled tumor growth.

HER-2 amplification has significant impact on treatment decisions related to breast cancer.

There are two tests for HER-2:

IHC (ImmunoHistoChemistry) and FISH (Fluorescence in situ Hybridization).

The IHC test looks at the protein on the surface of the cell by staining the cell with an antibody. The protein on the surface of the cell can be affected by tissue formalin fixation onto the slide. This can cause inaccurate interpretation of IHC results. In addition, IHC testing is subjective: the reader must judge the degree of color change in the cell against a non-standardized chart.

The fluorescence in situ hybridization test (FISH) is more accurate and reliable. It is good for all kinds of tissue: fresh, frozen, and formalin fixed, paraffin embedded tissue. It is also good for stored formalin fixed paraffin embedded tissue samples too. The FISH test measures HER-2 gene abnormality at the stable DNA level. The FISH test "paints" the HER-2 genes inside the cell, so they may be accurately counted. (National Cancer Institute: NIH.gov)

As I read the words, I started to understand the significance of the test and again I began to pray in earnest. *Please God, let the FISH test confirm that I DON'T NEED CHEMO!*

Date: Friday, 1-9-04
To: My Prayer Group
Subject: Metamorphosis - Part IV: Update
"Blessed are those who can give without remembering and take without forgetting" —Elizabeth Bibesco
Greetings to all and a Happy New Year!!!

I have had several people email me to ask why I haven't sent any updates...I am wondering if they miss them? Ha!!!!

Well, a few things have occurred that might be of interest...

First, I am doing very, very well...have been to the gym a few times this week, which has been quite inspirational in of itself.

I have had conversations with many people who "missed" me and I am realizing on a daily basis that I have been thrust into a "club" to which many members belong. Along with this membership, I have been given the opportunity to open myself spiritually and to share that with many others. Divine intervention continues to occur and I am always amazed at the results.

Last Sunday, some 24-year old kid hit the rear end of my car while I was sitting at a Stop/Right-hand turn lane...so, I have been dealing with that. I am going through his (dad's company) insurance because he hit me with the company van.

Although, I felt a significant "jolt" and have had some symptoms in my neck, I am praying that Celebrex will take care of those and that will be the end of it.

As far as I am concerned, I say: "That's it! —my "things that happen in three's" should be complete. MOVE ON to the next person!!!!" Yikes!

Next, let me tell you that TODAY is the LAST day of my 10-month vacation. I start work on Monday with Kelson Pharmacy, which is a pediatric specialty pharmacy based in Miami.

I am most happy about this, because I am back in the realm of my first love in nursing—pediatrics. I have accepted a Regional Sales Manager position, covering the territory from Tampa/St. Pete north to Gainesville/Jacksonville. To those of you that live in those areas, perhaps we can have lunch when I am in your city!!!

The company is only 2 years old, so there is alot of room for growth; and business development is a passion of mine.

So, as you can see, my novena to the Blessed Mother worked and She saw to it that not only did I get a job, but it is the RIGHT job for me...one in which I can provide service doing the things that I love!!

Lastly, because I am going to Miami for orientation next week, I had to reschedule my appointments for my next plastic surgeon "pump up" and the oncologist—moved from next week to the following week. Therefore, I won't have any updates on the FISH test and the impending chemo treatments until after the appointment on the 21st.

Please know that I am at peace and feel the joy of my metamorphosis...a rebirth...a new beginning. I am grateful to, and love all of you for your continued prayers and support.
Till the next update...
Love and light, Carla

Carla:
Sounds like things are going great! Your job sounds FAB!
Is it OK that you are back at the gym so soon? Guess you got the permission from the doctor.
Sorry about your car crash. That is always a bummer (getting the cars fixed, etc, etc.)
You know I ALWAYS love to hear the updates—especially with such good news! I am SO thankful things are going as they are for you!!!
Love, Sharon

Carla...
I am so thrilled to hear that all is proceeding well with your recovery...wow, workin' out?—you go girl! Sounds like you will be ready for another massage from my therapist, Joann. Let me know. Trish

Carla~
Sounds like you've got your new wings and are flying! Whatta great sight! Congrats on your new job! I just think it's

awesome that you landed such a perfect gig; it sounds perfect for you with room to grow. And, you get to work out of your house (which I love). You certainly deserve all of it

I do have a question for you. My ex-sister in law, who lives in Colorado, was just diagnosed with breast cancer (she got her biopsy results Monday). I honestly don't know what kind of support network she has going, but I do know that she has been under a great deal of stress as her father is living with her. Her kids are a great support to her. I don't know if she is open to talking with anyone about it, but, I thought I would ask you first if you would be willing to talk with her. Let me know your thoughts.

Continue to take good care Let's have lunch—see you soon.

Love, Sue

One of my friends, who was a former manager of mine, sent me a beautiful prayer card, stating that masses were being said each day on my behalf. Pat D. had experienced her own grief only a year earlier, when her husband died suddenly. It was astonishing to me—yet very heartwarming—that she could set aside her own grief and comfort me.

Date: January 19, 2004
Dear Pat~
Thank you for the card enrolling me in the Lourdes Prayer League and the Mass celebrated in my name each month at the Shrine of Our Lady of Lourdes in France and each day at the National Shrine of Our Lady of the Snows in Belleville, Illinois. Having recently experienced your own life-changing event, I am grateful for your empathy regarding this challenge that I am facing and the friendship and support that you offer.
Love~
Carla

After ten months of unemployment, the breast cancer diagnosis, the mastectomies and the speedy recovery, I was obviously on a "high" for a month or so. I started my new job on January 12th and went to Miami for a 3-day orientation. A week later, I went to see Dr. Molthrop to discuss the results of the FISH test.

I was sitting in the exam room reading a magazine, anxious to get through this appointment when Dr. Molthrop walked in.

He greeted me with that cute "little boy smile" and apologized for the confusion about the last appointment.

Walking over to the end of the room, Dr. Molthrop began to write on a white board that was apparently placed on the wall for teaching purposes...or to make a point.

He started by writing on the board: 1cm - +

"Your tumor was 1 centimeter, which is small—that's good!" He proclaimed, as he drew a circle around the plus sign.

"You had bilateral mastectomies—also good", as he drew another plus sign with a circle around it.

"You had no cancer in your lymph nodes" Another plus sign.

"BUT..."

Okay, here it comes.

"Your cancer is HER2Neu positive—that's not good." As he drew the negative sign and circled it, my nursing instincts kicked in and I knew this was not going in the direction I had hoped.

Dr. Molthrop continued, "Your FISH test was positive and that's not good." Again, he drew a negative sign with a circle around it.

"Even though you have 3 positives and 2 negatives", he said, "the best oncologist in the United States would say that you should have chemotherapy...just to be sure."

At this point, he was looking at me, sitting across the room, and he could see the disappointment in my eyes. He started giving me statistics and validation for the reasons as to why I should have chemo, but I wasn't listening.

I knew that he wouldn't recommend it if he didn't think it was necessary. But, for the past month, I really believed that I would not have to endure chemotherapy. I just felt drained.

My new boss, Nathan, had scheduled a strategic planning meeting the next day in Miami. I was going to meet the CEO, the CFO and a Vice President of the Practice Management division of the company. My bags were already packed and in the trunk of my car, so when I left Dr. Molthrop's office, I headed straight to the airport. My mind was dizzy with questions.

How can I start a new job and have chemotherapy at the same time?

How am I going to tell Nathan? Surely, he will think that I knew all along that I was going to need chemo.

This is my second week of work...how am I going to break the news—with all of the "head honchos" around?

I have to tell him—but when?

I was slowly spiraling into a major funk. I could think of nothing else during the 45-minute plane trip to Miami, the taxi drive to the hotel, or during dinner. When I got back to my room, I tried to divert my attention by watching television.

I finally fell asleep at about midnight. However at 3:00am, I awoke with the thought of chemotherapy on my mind and I couldn't go back to sleep. Three hours later, I dragged myself out of bed and into the shower. *Chemotherapy? First, I lose my breasts, now I am going to be bald! I cannot believe this!*

Our meeting was being held in the hotel conference room, so a few minutes before 8:00 am, I stepped into the elevator. It was a long way down to the second floor.

I sat in the conference room for about ten minutes, pacing the floor, waiting for my new employers to come through the door. At 8:15am, they all walked in, with bright smiles and sunny dispositions. *It's too bad I don't feel the same emotions.*

Promptly, at 8:30am, the CEO began the meeting, and with only 3 hours of sleep and a heavy mind, I sat through eight agonizing hours of questions, strategizing and planning for the new business that I was expected to bring to the company. The day seemed to drag on and on.

Finally at 5:00pm, with no opportunity to say anything about the chemo, I said goodbye to Nathan and jumped into the car with the CEO and CFO, who offered to drop me off at the airport.

The next few days were spent talking with family about my dilemma. Although they tried to cheer me up, I had a difficult time accepting the fact that I had to go through the process of chemotherapy...all while I was starting a new job.

Chemo...nausea...hair loss. Please God, help me wrap my mind around the fact that I need to go through this.

It took a few days, but I finally came to the place, where I knew I had to proceed and that everything would work out. My prayers, again, were answered.

> Sent: Friday, January 23, 2004
> To: My Prayer Group
> Subject: Metamorphosis: Phase V - Chemotherapy
> *He is a man of sense who does not grieve for what he has not, but rejoices in what he has.* —Epictetus
>
> Okay, it has taken a few days to come to grips with this, but on Wednesday, I was told that I have to go through chemotherapy. Bummer!!

On Wednesday morning, at the plastic surgeon's office, I was "pumped up"—and that afternoon, at the Oncologist's office, when Dr. Molthrop told me I needed to have chemo—I felt like the air was being let out of my balloon. *Boo-hoo!!*

Enough of that, though. God has listened to our prayers... but on this one, he just said: "No."

Of course, with a metamorphosis, you have to go into the cocoon stage—I guess I was hoping to bypass that, but that is not how it works in the Universe. So, into my cocoon I shall go (not literally, mind you—I am not putting my head in the ground. I will continue the need to surround myself with friends and family) awaiting the beautiful butterfly phase.

As we speak, I am wearing one of my two wigs (the one that is a little longer than the other—we call it my "weekend party hair") just to begin the "bonding process". The lady who sold me the wigs at Deborah's Divas suggested that I begin to "make friends" with it (she too, had cancer about 11 years ago.) I guess I will soon understand why my family name is Baldwin (get it?? "Bald one").

As far as the details, I can only tell you that if you read my last email on Wednesday, Dr. "Gorgeous" Molthrop pretty much affirmed what Dr. Z had to say at my last appointment; except that, since the HER2Neu and FISH test were positive, research indicates that EVEN THOUGH my tumor was only 1 cm, and I had the mastectomies, and my nodes were negative, the FISH is a predictor of aggressive cancer activity. So, IF I have any cells floating around this skinny little body, the chemo would wipe them out.

So, I began listening to my "Chemotherapy" visualization and affirmation CD and move forward from here. In the CD, it describes the chemo as a "golden healing liquid" that showers over me. One of the affirmations that I love is: "I thank the cancer cells for teaching me what I needed to learn. YOU CAN GO now!"

Although, Dr. Molthrop provided me with the "opportunity" to be in a 3-armed randomized clinical trial (for you laymen, that means there are 3 different types of treatment—one being the standard treatment and the other two include the standard treatment with an added NEW drug that is being researched called Herceptin. Randomized means that you are picked at random to be entered into one of the arms), I have decided that I will forego the trial—mainly because I am not guaranteed that I will get the new drug and secondly, even if I did, that treatment takes over a year—plus the Herceptin is given EVERY week for a year. So, I am opting for the 4 month treatment regimen, where I will get Adriamycin and Cytoxan four times (once every 2 weeks) and then 4 more treatments of Taxotere (once every 2 weeks)...for a total of 8 treatments.

I started my new job on Monday the 12th and received my first check yesterday. Halleluiah! I have yet to tell my boss that his new employee, although she doesn't have cancer anymore, must undergo chemotherapy. I thought I would wait until next Tuesday, when I see him face-to-face, thinking maybe I will wear my wig to show him that he won't even know that I am bald. Of course, the missing eyebrows and eyelashes may be a clue. Life is such an adventure! If he starts to cry, I may have to look for a new job; otherwise, I keep on working and try to schedule everything so it doesn't affect my work life—although, I am sure it is going to affect my social life. (Do you think my big, perky breasts will offset the bald head???—I know how my male friends would answer THAT question...you pervs!)

Oh yeah, I also need to have a port placed for the chemo to be administered directly into a LARGE vein (somewhere on my chest). I don't have a clue where Dr. Willard is going to place it. There is no fat on my chest whatsoever, so I am sure you will be able to see it when, and if, I wear a bathing suit or strapless dress. It will look like a giant button under my skin. I guess I will have to write on it." If you want to turn me on—press here!"

Well, that's it for this email. Nothing will happen until February 6th, when I have a MUGA Scan (WHO comes up with these names?), which is a test that looks at how effectively my heart is pumping (will they even FIND a heart??), because there is potential for the chemo to affect heart function. The following Monday, the 9th, I meet with Dr. Gorgeous and get the details of when I start the chemo.

Oh yeah, somewhere in between, I need to schedule surgery for the port placement and of course, work, eat and sleep.

So, ONCE AGAIN, I am asking you to keep me in my prayers; specifically that the chemo does its job without any complications and few side effects (none would be nice).
Lots of LOVE, Carla

Hi Carla...

Just thinkin' about you. Sounds like you are gearing up for the chemo—whatta process. Have you begun to listen to the chemo CD? If the CD doesn't feel quite right for you let me know, I have a friend in California who is certified in guided imagery and she may know of another tool.

In the meantime, I am surrounding you in white light! Let me know the date you begin chemo and I'll put a call into the Sisters, so they can pray for you. I also spoke to my massage therapist and she suggested waiting for her healing massage post chemo. She did think a long foot rub might be good therapy for you during this process, though. Take care of yourself and thanks for keeping me in the loop. Love, Sue

Well, Carla

The saga/challenge/opportunity continues. The Epictetus comment reminds me of my favorite quote from Henrik Ibsen "Nothing is...but what is not".
BRW

Carla:

As usual, a very good and positive update!

My friend Connie has diabetes and has to wear a pump in her bra all the time. It is about the size of a cell phone. I made her several feminine, lace-edged covers for the pump, so the plastic wouldn't rub against her skin. She's adjusted very well to the inconvenience and discomfort.

It's amazing what we can handle, get used to, and ignore, when we have to, isn't it? Such is life, I suppose. If it weren't so difficult, I guess they would call this heaven!!

I love you and continue to be in awe, dear friend...Trish

Hi Carla,

I am so glad you are keeping us updated. Craig and I are both keeping you in our thoughts and prayers.

If you ever need someone to take you to chemotherapy or need someone to sit with you during the treatment, please know that Craig has offered. If I am here, I would be happy to help. The really nice thing for Craig is that he is here during the week when some of your other friends may have a harder time getting off work... so don't hesitate to call.

While I was on my cruise last week, Craig got a call that his skin biopsies were positive for basil cell carcinoma. We are very grateful that is all it is, however it does mean he has to have them all removed. I felt terrible I wasn't here when he got that call... but he has done fine.

Please be sure to call if we can help in any way.
Take care,
With love, Jo

Car~

This last email was beautifully written as all the previous Metamorphosis chapters have been. Dark humor acerbically sprinkled between the painful lines...but in my mind, I can see your facial expressions. Maybe your next career should be a writer. But I am not talking in the near next. You have enough on your plate for now!

Ask about Zofran for the nausea, my sister Kathy says it is incredible. She took care of kids before they started using it, and she said there is such a dramatic difference in tolerance of treatment. But then, with your spiritual approach, you may not have ANY side effects. We will all aim for that one!

~Luv ya, Maur

Carla,

I was just thinking about you earlier, realizing that I haven't had an update in a while. I am so sorry about the chemo. I wish you didn't have to go through that. I know the chemo will probably wear you down so I would like to offer you any help I can with meals, running errands, etc. I really mean that, so don't be shy about asking!

How is your new job going? It sounds like it's perfect for you. I hope your boss takes the chemo news okay. If there is anything I can do for you, please let me know.

We really love you and will keep praying, praying, praying for you! Love, Jacqueline

We are praying for you and thinking about you. Let me know if you need anything
love you, debi

My Dear Carla,

God has asked a lot from you, and you have risen to his demands. I pray for your continued strength through these many months to come. If only we could wish away the things that devastate our lives—but wishing is a waste of time. We have to do what we must to survive. Please know that I am with you in spirit and support. Keep the faith.

Love, Pat D.

Carla,

Your brother is out of town and I just read your email. I am sorry that you have to go through chemo. You certainly have a great attitude and that means so much.

Of course, my prayers are always with you. I have a firm belief that you will be watched over.

It is also wonderful that you have such good friends. I am sure they will be as supportive throughout your chemo as they were for your surgery.

I'm glad the job is going well. Take care.

Love, Mercedes

As I pondered the emails, I thought about the upcoming year and all of the challenges that lay ahead. Of one thing, I was certain. The "old" Carla that existed previous to this experience was gone...and a "new" Carla was evolving.

8. Trying To Stay Balanced

*'For a long time it seemed to me that real life was about to begin, but there was always some obstacle in the way. Something had to be gotten through first; some unfinished business...then life would begin. At last it dawned on me that these obstacles **were** my life.'* —Bette Howland

Divine Intervention never fails to amaze me. Throughout this period, when I was feeling in a funk, something or someone would get my attention and provide me with some wisdom. Wisdom for embracing life and finding the balance that I needed to move forward on this tightrope called cancer.

On a rare, but particularly depressing day, I opened my email to find that one of my friends sent me the quote from Bette Howland (above); along with the following three questions:

> 1. How often do we miss the fullness of each day because we are fantasizing about some distant "green pasture" beyond our current struggles?
> 2. How often, in the face of challenges, are we unable to bring our best thinking to bear because we are impatiently trying to "fast forward" to a solution in the interest of "fixing" things?
> 3. How often are we so anxious to get through the obstacles so we can get on with our real purpose in life, that we fail to recognize that maybe, just maybe, the real purpose is in front of us?

How often? Much more than we want to admit.
The email continued:

> "For this week, may we move toward, not away from, the obstacles and difficulties with a fresh perspective. May we be blessed with a new resolve to **grow** through them...rather than just **go** through them. May we see in them the life they hold for us...today!"

As I read the email, the words touched me. For some odd reason, my mood was lightened as I felt that I was being "spoken to". These words were pertinent not only to my life, and what I was going through, but pertained to everyone I knew. We

all suffer challenges that must—at some point—be met and overcome.

A vivid memory was being recreated, as I thought about our life's purpose. Years before, I had attended a lecture by Harold Kushner[4], and I remember then, being enlightened by his words, as he expressed his thoughts related to the purpose of life. It was a quote I loved so much that a friend embroidered the words on a piece of cloth and had it framed for me. It is still hanging on a wall at home where I can see it daily:

"The purpose of life is not to win; the purpose of life is to grow."

Being re-awakened to this notion, I felt compelled to share the email with my prayer group—asking those three important questions. As I knew they would be, the responses were thoughtful and caring.

> Hello Carla,
>
> I liked the message you sent and I do think it is a very common attitude among all of us!!! I have a firm belief that there is growth only when we are faced with obstacles...we don't think we need God when everything is going well.
>
> ...I love my personal growth...what I mean is that I am so glad that I am able to grow and see beyond the challenges...to embrace them and then be thankful for the difficulty that resulted in growth. Of course, experiencing difficulty is somewhat easier when one has faith.
>
> I am sorry that you have to have the chemo...but thankfully they have something for your cell type...we want that cancer to stay gone!!!!
>
> Glad to hear about your job...it is so good to be busy, to enjoy what you are doing and to also get a paycheck!!!!
> Take care. You are continually in my prayers.
> Love, Olga
>
> Carla,
>
> I hope this note finds you in great spirits and with great expectations!! It has been so good to chart the course of your challenges with you through your emails—the next best thing to being with you personally. I hope you continue to know that I am thinking of you and wishing you success in all these things that are on your plate right now.
>
> The news about your job was good to hear—you sound very happy about it...Yay!

I walked Sabino Canyon this morning with a friend that is struggling with life issues—at almost 40, whether to have a kid or not (glad I'm not facing that one!), whether to change careers or not, whether to trade in her mate or not...whether to get up in the morning or not.

At almost 51 and a little further down the road, I think about how we all ask questions at each stage of our lives—sometimes due to necessity and sometimes just because we *can* (ask these questions). Michael calls them "luxury problems"—as we are not having to decide how to feed or shelter our body today with the knowledge that we will have the very same struggle again tomorrow (like most of my clients).

You may have a perspective borne of serious illness that gives you some freedom from this continual searching...but then, I think you have always had a mighty faith that things are as they need to be, and that the cerebral struggle to define destiny for ourselves is a lot of wasted energy.

Life on the home front is pretty sedate right now (please, Ms. God, don't make me pay for that statement!!). Looking forward to your next round of good news...Love, Beth

I had many friends that continually fed me the spiritual "vitamins" that I needed during this experience, which can be gleaned from the emails that are reproduced throughout this book.

Trish, (although she probably doesn't know it) was responsible for my own spiritual awakening so many years ago. She is an extremely creative person and a very talented writer. In the mid-90's, she used to have "journaling workshops"— several of which I attended. Through the journaling and my personal writings, I experienced many "breakthroughs" in my own spiritual development.

In order to continue the evolvement of her own spirituality, Trish reads publications that are enlightening and integrates the information into her own life. She also willingly and lovingly shares anything that can relate to others, as we all try to "make sense" of the challenges that life places in front of us. Trish, as you can see, was excited about sharing the following information with me.

Carla,
YOU MUST GET THIS BOOK by Mark Nepo. "The Book of Awakening"! He begins by talking about a wheel with the

spokes pointing outward to our individual uniqueness and pointing inward to our combined wholeness. He goes on to say:

"Not surprisingly, like most people, in the first half of my life, I worked very hard to understand and strengthen my uniqueness. I worked hard to secure my place at the rim of the Wheel and so defined and valued myself by how different I was from everyone else. But in the second half of my life, I have been humbly brought to the center of the Wheel, and now I marvel at the mysterious oneness of our spirit.

Through cancer and grief and disappointment and unexpected turns in career—through the very breakdown and rearrangement of the things I have loved—I have come to realize that, as water smoothes stone and enters sand, we become each other. How could I be so slow? What I've always thought set me apart binds me to others.

Never was that more clear to me than when I was sitting in a waiting room at Columbia Presbyterian Hospital in NY City, staring straight into this Hispanic woman's eyes, she into mine. In that moment, I began to accept that we all see the same wonder, all feel the same agony, though we all speak in a different voice. I know now that each being born, inconceivable as it seems, is another Adam or Eve."

Carla, I felt like he was talking about **your** experience and the reality of what you've been through. I think you'd like this book as much as I do! Luv, Trish

After reading this email, I began to reflect on the unexpected turns in my own life. I felt like I was on a "fast-forward mode" of continual growth—trying to balance the activities of my (real) daily life with the surreal experience of cancer that I was also living.

My new job was progressing smoothly and I soon had the opportunity to talk with Nathan about the chemotherapy. After all of the anxiety that this situation produced, I found that Nathan considered it to be a "non-issue". He had recently lost his own mother to cancer and he was extremely sensitive to the emotional turmoil that I was undergoing. He expressed his support and approval by saying, "I found the right person for this job. The only concern I have about you going through chemo is that you will work too hard—promise me that when you get tired, you will take it easy. You are going to be fine."

Was this the oneness of spirit that Mark Nepo had described?

Along with the information about Nathan's response, I sent the group an email, with a suggestion to buy the *Book of Awakening*.

> Carla...
> What a wonderful book suggestion! Mark Nepo is full of rich observations (and a man who has faced his own trials through cancer). Thanks for the update. I am so glad it went well with Nathan, what a gift (and relief...I'm sure) It just means you've landed in a good spot.
> I will keep you in my prayers this week, sending lots of light your way. Love, Sue
>
> Hi Carla,
> This last email you sent with the section from Mark Nepo's book, I found to be so refreshingly true.
> I hope all goes well with your chemo and you are blessed with no side effects. You know that what you are experiencing could be any of us. I am glad for your new blessings and I am always amazed at how much growth comes from something untoward. Why do we grow the most in adversity? I think that is how God works...
> Your friend, Olga

All work and no play has never been my philosophy. I have always felt the need to maintain a sense of balance between my work life and my home life. Six weeks after my surgery, I was feeling great and ready to socialize. So, Trish and I decided to go out and celebrate my 'first venture out of the house'.

After arriving home a little after midnight, I wrote a quick email to my sister, who had called me earlier that evening and encouraged me to go out.

> Sent: Saturday, January 24, 2004 12:09 AM
> Subject: Good nite...
> Bunnie~
> Sorry I didn't get to talk with you too long this evening. I really appreciate the calls that you make while "stuck in Chicago traffic". I DID go out dancing with my friend, Trish tonite. I wore my leather pants and my snakeskin jacket and boots. I had SEVERAL people come up and tell me how FABULOUS I looked...men and women! I had a lot of fun and was glad I went. Talk to you soon. I love you!
> Fabulous and Forever 47

> Carla~
> You ARE fabulous! I'm glad you went out. Now, we have
> to get Cookie "back into the game!"
> I'm sorry about the chemo future. But, I know that you
> are handling it. The prayers and good thoughts will
> continue to pour your way.
> I love you — JanJan/Bunnie

My birthday is January 29th...I have always LOVED my
birthday. Most years I would start the celebration on January
1st, providing my friends with a countdown of "shopping days"
until my birthday. For the past ten years, I have celebrated my
birthday with Diana, whose birthday falls on January 31st.
Anytime we had a party, it would be "theme-oriented" and we
would invite 40-50 people. There were "Black Tie" parties (where
you could wear anything—as long as you wore some type of
black tie), toga parties, and the most popular: Pajama parties
(where everyone wears lounge wear).

However, this year, I wasn't in the partying mood—at least
not in the mood for a *big* party. I did want to share my birthday
and celebrate with my close friends, though. So, with very little
fanfare, about 14 of us gathered at a local restaurant; and
Diana and I once again celebrated our birthdays together...this
time with a slightly different theme—one that incorporated my
attitude about going through the treatment for breast cancer.

It turned out to be a fun time with lots of laughter and great
conversation. Although it wasn't one of our infamous pajama
parties, we all had a wonderful time. After dinner, several of us
even went out dancing!

Personally, I found it to be a great way to stay balanced and
prepare for the next phase of my treatment.

The morning after my celebration, I checked my emails and
had a few that included birthday wishes...

> Carla~
> I sent off a birthday card to you today—late, I know...and
> when searching for stamps I found some not so exciting, run-
> of-the-mill flag stamps along with my 'fund-the-fight' stamps
> and I thought "how appropriate!" So, I attached two to the
> envelope, and then saw that the words 'breast cancer' were
> prominent on the top of them. I thought "Oh no! What a
> mistake to make such a loud statement, when Carla surely

doesn't need any reminders!" I tried to peel them off.....and then thought: "How ridiculous! Just send the damn thing so she gets it."

Isn't it interesting how serious illness affects one's behavior toward others...Is it because the small things are usually what we can control, and we want to get it RIGHT??! I'm sure you have stories to tell of many a faux pas, or awkward moments made worse over a totally inconsequential thing. So, if you are offended by my stamps...TOO BAD!!!!!

Love you, kiddo, and hope your course through the mine field is accompanied by fair weather and birds singing...
Beth

Carla~

Please know I'm with you EVERY STEP of the way! Let me know your chemo schedule, so I can take you or pick you up. I WANT TO BE A PART OF IT ALL. We're connected at the hip, you know!

I so loved your birthday and life celebration! And I'm so glad you are my dear, dear friend.
Your OLDEST and one of your DEAREST friends,
Trish

Keeping balanced also means keeping your perspective on life and maintaining a sense of humor. I couldn't resist sharing this email with my prayer group.

Sent: Thursday, February 05, 2004
To: My Prayer Group
Subject: If the shoe fits...
Today is International Day of The Very Good Looking, Beautiful and Damn Attractive People, so send this message to someone you think fits this description. Please do not send it back to me as I have already received over fifty thousand messages and my inbox is jammed.
Carla

Of course, I could count on my friends to keep me balanced...by treating me as they always had!

Car~
Excuse the rest of us uglies of the world...but we do congratulate YOU!
Have a nice day. Maur

9. Preparing for Chemo

'Ills of the body may be cured by physical remedies or by the power of the spirit acting through the soul.'

— Paracelsus, Father of Modern Medicine

To: "My Prayer Group"
Sent: Tuesday, February 10, 2004
Subject: Metamorphosis - Part VI: The Downhill Slide
Greetings to my favorite Prayer Group~

The saga continues and I am ready for the next phase of this challenge called cancer.

Many, many wonderful things have happened over the past three months *(yes, it has been 3 months since this all started)*. I am grateful to all of you for your continued prayers and support...and your awareness that I still need assistance from my family and friends; and I thank God every day that you are in my life.

As many of you know, I had my port (for chemo administration) placed during an outpatient treatment last Friday. Kelly drove me to the hospital and planned to take me home; however, the surgery was delayed, so she had to leave for a horse show after they wheeled me into the Operating Room. Take heart, though—my back-up nurse, Nadine, was kind enough to pick me up and drive me home and then made a scrumptious dinner for me.

I was surprised that I had more soreness with this surgery than with the mastectomies—most likely because the port was placed on my right clavicular area and any shoulder movement caused a pulling sensation. Surgery went well, though. My infamous surgeon, Dr. Sarah Willard (she's the BEST!), said I did GREAT.

I asked her to "talk to me" while under anesthesia...to say things like: "Your chemo will go well...outcome will be good...you will be ravenously hungry and will have no nausea." The nurse anesthetist told me that Dr. Willard talked to me the whole time! She also attached a white sticker beside my port and wrote: "For a good time, press here (with an arrow pointing to the port, which looks like a button).I can't remove it either, because they placed a large Tegaderm (clear plastic dressing) over it, which won't be removed until I have chemotherapy.

Soooooooo, of course, Dr. Gorgeous saw it!!! —(for a picture of him, go to the following website:

98

http://www.orlandooncology.com/molthrop.) He is pretty straight-laced, so I don't think he was amused, although, he knows what a maniac Dr. Willard is. (*I love her!*)

Yes, I saw Dr. Molthrop yesterday and had a gazillion questions for him, the most important of which were: can I exercise, can I take herbal supplements, can I have massages, can I have an occasional glass of wine, should I take Co-Q 10??? YES, no, yes, NO, no.

He told me that last night was the last night I should have wine, since I am starting chemo on Friday. So-o-o, guess what?! I decided I am giving up wine for Lent!

Dr. Molthrop actually wanted me to start my chemo right after my appointment yesterday afternoon and I said: "NO...*I wasn't planning* on that. Besides my only brother is in town from Hotlanta and he invited me to dinner."

I left the office and headed for the Westin Grand Bohemian (one of THE NICEST hotels and BEST restaurants in Orlando) where I had suggested my brother meet me. I had 2 glasses of Pinot Noir and a fabulous dinner AND dessert (I considered it my "Last Supper").

Thank you, Bro, for the wonderful dinner and the fabulous conversation! Your visit was an unexpected surprise and what I consider another Divine Intervention. For the record, your comment about my looking like Dolly Parton was not appreciated.

By the way, the results from my MUGA scan (which stands for Multi-gated Analysis—and measures the pumping efficacy of the heart) were excellent!! So, I move forward with the Adriamycin and Cytoxan, for 4 treatments, starting on Friday the 13th. I thought that was an appropriate date to start—as it is a date which will live in infamy in my mind.

Trish will be taking me to and from treatment (Kelly has a horse show, of course) and Marge will come with jammies and slippers in hand, and will spend the night at my house this weekend in case there are any "after effects". With friends like this, can I be any more blessed???

Work is going great. I have been employed for one month...and things are going swimmingly! I have had a few big ticket referrals, so I am a hero in the mind of my boss, Nathan. Of course, once Kay's office starts to refer, my numbers will go off the charts!!!

My hair is getting longer than I care to admit, but I just can't see paying for a haircut/highlight at this late stage. To Judy (my hairdresser): I want you to know that I have been chopping the top a little (I know how she HATES when I do that, but in a few weeks, it really won't matter). Trish insists that she likes my hair darker with just a few wisps of blonde, so I am considering keeping it that way after it grows back; however, who knows what color it will be when it grows back??!!.

Well, I must go eat...it's 8pm and I need to keep some meat on these bones. Anyone who knows of some high calorie, low fat recipes, I would love to have them.

Til the next time. LOVE and LIGHT to all.

Carla

Car-

Oh what a hoot! I guess they recognize a good time when they see it. I am glad that it went well for you. One more step on this long, but successful journey. I continue to offer prayers for your continued strength. You are the best...next to me, of course.

Luv ya, Maur

Hi Carla!

Thanks for the updates—they are one of the ONLY reasons I even sit down at this piece of machinery. One of these days I'll take a computer class!

We were so happy to hear about your new position—it was up there with all of the things for you that we have been praying about. I am truly not surprised that you have won them over.

Now, as far as your chemo etc. and your hair—what happened to that idea that I (you know, YOUR HAIRDRESSER) was going to cut your hair into a really cute short, short cut—then when needed, cut it down to finger length or buzz it? I would love to do that for you!! Of course, it's on me!!

If you are worried about it being all dark, I could always put a few wisps of blonde through the front, as Trish said. Don't know what your doc would say about your getting highlights; I wouldn't want it to fall out before it's time. Anyway, you get the drift!!

Just ask the *professional* (in case you don't know who that is—of course that would be ME)!

Lots of love,

Judy

P.S. Thank you for sharing Dr. Gorgeous' picture with us! Is he married?

Car~

No wine? YIKES! Oh well, I usually give it up for Lent too...and it is doable.

The thoughts about your hair sound interesting, so I cannot wait to see what the outcome is.

As to work, congrats on your fast start out of the gate and we both know your company could not have done better.

This next phase probably is the toughest, but you have been working your way up to it. What are your pre-meds for the chemo treatment? Ask for Zofran!

The prayers and thoughts continue your way, and will be intensified on Friday.

Love Maur

Carla/Darla/Mimi:

...whatever you are calling yourself these days. Thank you for the updates. I love that you continue to have a sense of humor about yourself, your treatments and cancer. You are an inspiration to me.

I've started to forward your messages to Kristin (apparently, I wasn't doing that and she was a tad upset with me that she "wasn't in the loop" regarding her "auntie.")

Glad to hear that Uncle Beeeaaallll stopped by to see you. I just love when our brother "pops" into DC...to me those are the best visits (unexpected surprises...I LOVE SURPRISES!!!)

I'm going to do my best to get down there and check out the new and improved Carla. But in the meantime, please know that you are in my morning and night prayers (Come on St. Peregrine!!) as well as on the prayer cards of many people in my prayer circle. I'm trying to recruit some women from my office to team up with me for the AVON BREAST CANCER 2-day event in May...more on that later.

Gotta scoot.

I love you.

Ann

Dear Carla:

Omigosh, Dr. Gorgeous is GORGEOUS!! Did you say whether he's married or not? I'm so amazed by how young doctors are these days. They USED to all be OLDER than me! NOW, they're all BABIES! That's what I thought about Dr. Rotatori, when I met him in 1994. My gosh, that was 10 years ago. Where is my LIFE going??

By the way, I went shopping for my upcoming birthday party...and did I mention that my red dress was $19.99, my stilettos (Nine West) were $19.99, and my cream colored shawl was $6.99? The entire outfit, head to toe, was just over $50. I am such a GOOD shopper!! If I paid any less for them, the store would be paying ME to take them home! I told Sheila I'd have to take a second pair of shoes to the party with me just in case it was necessary for me to walk anytime during the evening! I'm really excited about this party! Can you tell??

Maybe we should go to a movie tomorrow night after work, or meet at Stonewood for a club soda. You need to do something social before you start chemo on Friday. Are you interested? Trish

Dear Carla –

Sorry I missed you when I called. I just wanted you to know that I light a candle for you (and Daddy and Karen) every Sunday. We are all praying for you.

Good luck on Friday. I wish I could be there in body, but you know my heart is with you.

I love you.

JanJan

Dear Carla,

I was hiking with a friend in the high upper reaches of Sabino Canyon this morning, and thinking of you. On the climb down, we rounded a corner to come face-to-face with a deer and her fawn. They regarded us warily, and then decided to continue munching on branches. We watched as they eventually picked their way down the slope and out of sight.

It reminded me of your trip here when we hiked up Cathedral Rock in Sedona—a very different encounter than the one with that hard-charging "Sedona spirit" we were so lucky to experience. But I continue to be in awe of the world that exists outside of my head and the usual day-to-day junk.

Friday the 13th looms...but it will be all right.

Love you, Beth

As I moved forward with my "Metamorphosis", I continued to research breast cancer and chemotherapy. One evening while I was going from website to website, I 'happened upon' (another Divine Intervention!) an article related to a book *The Message From Water*[5]. It was written by a Japanese scientist, Masaru Emoto, who came up with a theory that, when a water molecule crystallizes, *pure* water becomes *pure* crystal, but contaminated water may not crystallize as beautifully as pure water.

With his friend and colleague, Dr. Lee Lorenzen, Emoto also began to study the properties of water and how human thought/feeling can influence it.

Using High-speed photography, he found that crystals formed in frozen water reveal changes after specific, concentrated thoughts were directed toward it. Small amounts of water (an 8 oz. glass) as well as large areas of water (such as dams and lakes) were used in these experiments and in all cases the water samples reflected a molecular change.

Music and visual images were used to stimulate the water samples. The water was also exposed to words written on paper and photographs placed underneath or around the glass containers to see if these energies had any impact. **They did.**

His experiments were recorded in his book and illustrate the profound *power of sound and thought vibrations on water.*

Water from clear unpolluted springs and water that had been blessed or exposed to loving words showed brilliant, often complex and invariably beautiful snowflake patterns, sparkling with brilliant color and luminosity. By contrast, water from chemically treated sources, polluted waters or those exposed to negative thought forms, showed incomplete, asymmetrical patterns, low reflectivity and dull colors.

After reading this very interesting study, I decided that I was going to send positive energy into my chemotherapy infusion so that it would provide the best outcome possible as it ran through my bloodstream and into my tissues.

On Friday, the 13th, I arrived at the chemotherapy suite with Trish. The suite was a large treatment room with about 15 leather recliners lining the walls and a nurse's station in the middle. Each recliner had a straight wooden chair beside it—for the family member or friend who accompanied the patient.

I chose the recliner closest to the doorway, later wondering if my choice expressed an unconscious desire to run away from this whole experience. I looked around the room and observed the other patients who were either asleep in their recliners, reading a book or chatting non-stop with their companion sitting in the wooden chair. If I didn't know better, it could have been a scene at an airport, where people were waiting for their plane to arrive.

As I was getting comfortable, pulling out my magazines and preparing for the 2 hour treatment, the nurse came over and introduced herself.

"My name is Tosha and I will be taking care of you today," she said, while donning a pair of latex gloves. She then began to explain the procedure for my first and next three chemo treatments.

"Just relax", Tosha said gently, "this will feel like a bee sting", as she injected xylocaine into the skin over my chemo port. After a few minutes, she pushed a large needle through the skin and into the port. I felt the pressure of the needle puncturing through the rubber cap of the port, with a resounding "thump".

As she was attaching the IV tubing to the needle in the port, Tosha continued to explain. "Next, I will hang some antinausea medicines to drip into your IV. That will take about 20 minutes...then I will slowly push two syringes filled with Adriamycin into the IV; and finally, I will hang the Cytoxan, which will drip in over about 45 minutes." *Okay, I am as ready as I will ever be—let's do it!*

While the antinausea medicines were being administered, Tosha reviewed with me the side effects of which I should be aware while undergoing my chemotherapy treatments. I guess at that point, I was either overwhelmed or just not paying much attention... as I would learn a few weeks later.

Fifteen minutes passed and the IV bag with the nausea medicines was empty. Tosha brought over two huge syringes filled with red liquid. This was the dreaded Adriamycin— otherwise known as "red devil".

Prior to "pushing" the Adriamycin, Tosha offered me a cup of ice and told me to hold some ice in my mouth as I was receiving the Adriamycin. Cooling the mouth, she said, would help prevent mouth sores associated with this particular drug.

NOW I understand that scene in the "Sex and the City" episode where Samantha was getting chemotherapy and she, Charlotte, Carrie and Miranda were eating Popsicles!

As the nurse pushed in the Adriamycin, I could feel the cool medicine being introduced into my veins and I said a quick prayer that it would find any aberrant cancer cells and kill them with a vengeance!

Next came the final part of this day's treatment.

Prior to her hanging the Cytoxan, I wrote the words: LOVE, GRATITUDE on a post-it note, sent my intentions to the chemotherapy *to do its work*, and asked Tosha to attach the post-it to the IV bag. I thought she might think I was crazy for doing this, but without a word, she took the post-it note and attached it to the bag.

At that point, I knew that whatever beliefs I had, there would be no judgment from the nurses. And my plan was to do this with every treatment—with my positive and loving intentions expressed in the liquid medicines as they flowed through my veins—*doing what needed to be done.*

Sent: Sunday, February 15, 2004 7:18 PM
To: My Prayer Group
Subject: Metamorphosis - Part VII: Chemo Countdown
    One down and 7 to go...
    On Friday I went for my first chemo treatment— accompanied by my trusty friend, Trish. I guess I failed to prepare her for the procedure, because she arrived with no book (for the two hour treatment) and wore a sleeveless top with a wide knit sweater and no socks. It was quite cold in the treatment room, so when I asked the nurse for a blanket, I turned it over to Trish, who was shaking because she was so cold!
    The first treatment itself was pretty uneventful...the nurse put a needle into my port and dripped a small amount of IV fluid with Zofran and Decadron (to prevent nausea/vomiting), then pushed the Adriamycin over 5 minutes and then dripped the Cytoxan (with IV fluid) over about 45 minutes. I listened to my meditation/affirmation CD, while Trish took a nap in one of the lounge chairs. Then we went home—like I said, uneventful.
    My faithful friend, Marge, met us at my house—with suitcase in hand—in preparation for her weekend stay. We ate Thai food for dinner and, even though we were both exhausted, we stayed up until 11:00pm, so that I could take my Zofran (by mouth every 8 hours). I didn't sleep well that night, but that is not unusual these days for me. I woke at 1am, then 3am and stayed awake until about 4:30am, then got up at 7am—took another Zofran—and slept until 9:45am. Marge and I had breakfast and then sat around for a few hours and talked, when we decided to go for a walk.
    Right before we left, the phone rang—it was Phil (the guy I have been seeing)...asking how things went. As I was telling him, the doorbell rang and when I opened the door—there he was! Valentine's Day flowers in hand...and all I could think of was: "SHIT! I haven't showered and I have NO make-up on (he

hasn't seen me without makeup). I look like crap!" Oh well, I guess I am going to look even crappier soon!

After Phil left, Marge and I went for a long walk and then stopped in to see her sister and dad, who live in my neighborhood. After the visit, it was spitting rain, so we put up our umbrellas and headed home.

The afternoon was filled with phone calls from friends and well-wishers and at about 6:00pm, we decided to go out for barbeque ribs! Marge made an excellent date for Valentine's Day, but the weather was horrible!! We wanted to rent a funny movie, so we stopped at Blockbuster and rented Freaky Friday. We went to bed at about midnight and I basically had a repeat performance of the night before.

I am so grateful to Marge, that she gave up her weekend to spend it with her buddy. And I am thankful to Ed for loaning me his wife and giving up whatever romantic notions he had for Valentine's Day.

Today, I have just stayed in my robe, no nausea or vomiting—but no appetite to speak of. I have been just lounging and napping all day.

A little while ago, Kelly's friends, Michelle and Polette called to say they were dropping by—again no makeup and no shower! I ran in and put on some clothes *and my wig*, so I would look halfway presentable. When I told them I had on my wig, they were pretty shocked that they couldn't tell, so I guess it will pass for my hair for the next 6 months. According to the nurse, I should start to lose my hair in about two weeks, so those of you that wanted to see me bald need to make flight reservations to Florida within the next few months. For the rest of you, I will take pictures!

From this point forward, I will be having chemo every other week on Thursdays. Polette (whose mother recently finished chemo for breast cancer) advised me that I will definitely need someone to drive me back and forth to chemo...so, if you are available—just let me know and I will put you on the list. It's certainly an experience that you will long remember!

Until the next time, please keep me in your prayers and if you want to come over for dinner—call me—it may help my appetite to share a meal with my friends!!
Love to all, Carla

Hey Carla/Mimi –
I just picked up your last e-mail (after watching Sex and the City). I'm so sorry that you have to go through the chemo.

Some day you'll be standing up there, just like Samantha, tossing your wig to the world. I'll call you this week.
I love you. JanJan

Hey:
I cannot understand from the update whether you actually got through this OK, other than no appetite. Did the Zofran work?
I thought about you all weekend and prayed on Friday.
If I could drive you, I would. And being a Yankee, no one would have to worry about keeping me warm! I think it is prophetic that this guy (why have you not said anything about him before?) saw you without makeup. I thought NO ONE saw that!
God Bless and keep the faith when the hair starts coming out. What comes in might be very interesting (curly too)!
Love, Maur

The Zofran kept me from vomiting, but I just couldn't think about food without feeling somewhat queasy...and it would be a year before I could eat Thai food or barbeque ribs again.

Although I didn't know it at the time, I probably should not have eaten such rich foods right after having the chemo. I couldn't stand the smell...or the sight of either of those foods—both of which I loved. Don't ask me why...but it happened

Also, I was concerned about the problems that I was beginning to have with my sleep patterns. As I began to wonder about this, I received an email from a friend Patty, in Seattle, who had breast cancer treatment the year before me.

Carla,
Glad to hear that the first treatment was uneventful—sounds great. You are probably aware that it is the Decadron keeping you awake. I was always wired for at least two days from the Decadron.
And yes, as far as meals go, it is very helpful to have friends come over. I found myself with little appetite and feeling kind of crummy much of the time; but if I had a dinner guest, I would eat and feel better.
Sounds like things are very much under control and going well. It took my hair about 3.5 weeks to fall out—I suppose everyone is different.
Take Care.
Patty

Carla/Darla the Beautiful (that's your new name from me)...

I'm glad to hear that you tolerated the first chemo treatment well and I'm praying that the remaining therapies will go just as well. Your sleep patterns leave alot to be desired.

I'm thankful for your friends and Kelly's friends who have been transformed into "angels" and I pray for them everyday. I'm sure that they have made personal sacrifices to be with you and to be "there for you" and in my mind that says a hell of alot about their character and friendship.

And Janis' thoughtfulness and kind acts—I'm embarrassed that I haven't risen to the occasion like she has, but I am a work in progress and I'll "get there"... just please be patient with me.

Not much going on...I was talking to one of the guys at the gym about my trainer, and my diet etc. and as he was starting to leave, he comes back and says: "Without sounding forward or overly flirtatious, I need to tell you that I think you have an outstanding body—your workout routine is great—cause I watch you...and every time you walk into the gym—I think: "She looks great!"

OK, so it gets better...I was at Chico's, buying a sweater and I'm at the counter and the checkout clerk told me that I was beautiful...have a great complexion and color and she just loves my hair color (not blonde anymore....gone auburn and red...HOT like a devil woman...oooohh laa laa)

Again, I digress...

...and I'm thinking Wow! You made my day. I was walking on air. I've never had anyone pay compliments to me like that. I didn't know how to respond (except grin like a fool).

I guess this isn't very nice sharing this with you, considering what you are going through...and I don't mean to make you feel bad or anything like that. After all you are going to be the one with the beautiful boobs and face when you finish your treatments!! Then I'll really be envious!

I hope you have a great day and are able to find some beauty somewhere today...remember to give thanks!
I love you. Ann

Annie~

Why would I not want to hear that you are finally recognizing your own beauty? I think that is why we must face these challenges—there is always something to learn about ourselves. Just make sure that you BELIEVE IT...because it is true. You ARE beautiful—inside and out—but you don't need anyone or anything to confirm that for you...that you must do yourself.

I love you!...and NO apologies necessary from you—you have always stepped up to the plate with the ones you love. Carla/Darla/Mimi

Hi honey girl.

I only wish I could come cross country for dinner! It sounds like things are going pretty well so far. I don't like the sleeplessness though. You need your rest. Ask your doc for something to help. It's important to get quality sleep.

Yes, Marge is a gem and I'm so glad she's there for you during this "bump in the road." I guess I will get to see you sans hair when I come in May.

Also sounds like a nice guy lurking in the background. Most guys would high tail it to the hills. So keep him around for a while.

I hope and pray everything stays at an even keel, and that the physical ill-effects will stay at bay.

But do get something to help you sleep—it's pretty standard. Listen to your nurse!
Love and kisses, Prissy

Hey LaLa~

Glad to hear it's so far so good. Good idea to keep something in your stomach to avoid the nausea. You skinny bitch!!! You can't afford to lose any weight. I, on the other hand, could stand to ditch about 40 lbs. I get so bored in the evening—junk food is my downfall. You take good care of yourself!!
Prayers and Hugs—helen

Preparing for chemotherapy is an important step in the process of breast cancer treatment...physically, mentally, emotionally and spiritually.

Before and during treatment, I prepared myself by eating well and continuing to exercise (when I could). I even hired a trainer, so that I would have some motivation—albeit, forced motivation—to exercise when I really didn't want to. Amy, my trainer was experienced with chemotherapy patients, so she focused not only on a "lite" regimen of strength training, but also on core body strength so that I could maintain my activities of daily living. Many days, just walking into the gym gave me a sense of control and an inner strength that helped me through treatments that often made me feel so weak.

Emotionally, I prepared myself by listening to a guided meditation. Every night, I fell asleep listening to the Healing Journeys[2] "Chemotherapy" Meditation CD. I found it to be relaxing, yet powerful; because it suggested that the chemo was a "golden, healing liquid that surged through my body to get rid of the cancer cells". In my mind, this was certainly a better way to think about the chemo, rather than "a poison which kills the cells".

Intellectually, I knew I would have some reaction to the chemotherapy, but prior to having chemo, no one can know which physical side effects will rear their ugly head—not even the doctors, because everyone reacts differently. Therefore, it was important for me to do my research. After talking with many people who had gone through breast cancer treatment, I realized that I needed to know what the *possible* side effects were...only then would I know how they could be treated if they manifested in me. What I eventually realized was that *many side effects can be eliminated and most of them can be reduced.* But it is a matter of recognizing them early and asking for help in treating them. Basically, a side effect is a feeling or symptom that is not normal for you.

As most people do, I learned as I went along and recognized a little too late that I could have avoided some of the side effects of chemotherapy. Little did I know that the persistent feeling of nausea could be relieved by chewing Tums or Rolaids every 3 or 4 hours, or taking Pepcid or Zantac...or all of the above! I guess I felt that side effects were "normal" occurrences of chemotherapy to be tolerated. Well, guess what—if it makes you feel bad in any way—there is probably some remedy that will lessen or eliminate it. So, *insist upon finding out what that remedy is and take it!*

I know that my healthcare background provided some benefit while going through this experience; but overall, I was just another woman who was "trying to figure it all out as I went along".

"Googling" became a part of my everyday vocabulary. If I wanted to find out about new medications that were available to help alleviate side effects, I went to my computer and "googled" whatever I was feeling and the appropriate medications used to treat those symptoms. And then, I would be sure to ask the doctor for the medicine...and if that didn't work, I tried a different medication...*and I kept on asking*...so that I could avoid those "yucky" days and feel as good as possible while going through this treatment. At one point, I was taking SeaCure[6] for my queasiness ...and it worked! I highly recommend taking it at the beginning of any chemo that will cause nausea.

And, lastly, but most importantly, I prepared myself spiritually through prayer...and through the prayer of others. The power of prayer is amazing and I know that this experience would have been much more difficult without my faith in a Higher Power. So, *for me, that was the most powerful of all the preparation steps.*

10. Living through the Treatments

'Let us rise up and be thankful, for if we didn't learn a lot today, at least we learned a little, and if we didn't learn a little, at least we didn't get sick, and if we got sick, at least we didn't die; so, let us all be thankful.' —Buddha

Date: Wed, 03 Mar 2004
To: My Prayer Group
Subject: Metamorphosis - Part VIII: Chemo Countdown 2

One month down and 3 months to go (that sounds better than 2 treatments down and 6 to go).

Sorry that it took awhile to get this update to you, but I had a little rougher time this round. (I now understand why they call it "rounds of chemo"—it's very much like being in the boxing ring!)

Anyway, after 5 days of nausea and some advice from another breast cancer survivor (thanks Patty!), I have come to realize that I don't have to suffer with nausea at all...there are DRUGS to take care of it—which is what I told my Dr. Gorgeous from the beginning—GIVE ME THE DRUGS. Yes, this coming from someone who wouldn't take an aspirin for a headache prior to this experience.

However, apparently Dr. Gorgeous wanted me to ASK for them—which is what I did yesterday. Well, it was really more like DEMAND—but, you get the picture. I now have a prescription for Phenergan, which I will take with and after the Zofran (which I found out only works for the 72 hours that the chemo is in the system).

Alas, after going down to the office today to demand—I mean to discuss—my options, I found out that what I have been feeling is NOT from the chemo itself, but from the results of the chemo and its effect on my GI tract—increased stomach acid (which, of course, I have never experienced in my life, so I didn't know the feeling). The solution: an over-the-counter antacid, i.e. Tagamet, Zantac or Pepcid ...and Rolaids!!! (Yeah, that's what I said: "Are you freaking kidding me???") Note to Maureen: Please tell your patients about this BEFORE they have this absolutely UNNECESSARY experience.

Oh yeah, regarding the hair loss—it has begun. In fact, on day 15, the crown of my head felt sore, like I had been dragged through the cave by a Neanderthal man...and on day 17, my hair ended up in the shower drain—not all of it, but enough for me to say: "Ok, time to get my head shaved! " I know this will be a surprise to Judy, my faithful friend and hairdresser, who so generously cut my "do" only six days before—making me look like what Kelly called a brown-haired Sharon Stone (and what I thought looked like an Auschwitz survivor!).

Anyway, Judy's shop was closed on Monday, and I **had** to get it off, so at 11:30am on Monday, I went in to the hair salon near my house and at 11:33am, I walked out the door!!! Now I look like Sinead O'Connor (isn't she the one that tore up the pope's picture?)

I just want you to know that I have a beautifully shaped head and my face is "heart-shaped" (which I never knew) and VERY LITTLE gray hair---yes, it is about 1/8" and very brown (much to the chagrin of my younger, gray-but-dyed-brown-haired friends!! HA!)

I have been wearing my wig and actually made some sales calls with it on today, without incident. Of course, when I come home, the first thing I do is yank it off, much like I used to do with my bra.

Speaking of bras, I have had 500cc of saline injected into the expanders so far and Dr. Rotatori wanted to put another 50 cc in next week—but I called this morning and cancelled that appointment. I think I have been blown up enough. I look like a Mack truck's headlights when you see me coming head-on!!!

Work is going well...my boss called me today and told me that if we were keeping score, I was winning this week. Of course, my response was "I don't keep score, I am working for the TEAM". He liked that answer, but says the accountants want to know my score. (Damned accountants.)

Lastly, I am in the process of coming up with the top ten GREAT reasons for having chemotherapy. So far, I have five: (as Letterman would countdown)

10. You can save as much as $135 per month on highlights.

9. You don't have to buy shampoo and conditioner for at least 6 months.

8. You don't have to go through the excruciating pain of a bikini wax before summer swimsuit time.

7. You are a cheap date (no alcohol or dessert).

6. You are a cheap date (no appetite).

I am sure I will come up with the other five over the next few months; but if you have any you want to add, I will consider them when I publish my book. Oh yes, another Divine Intervention that I must tell you about. My dear, sweet Kelly has moved back in with me, due to circumstances beyond her control (roommate problems). But, as I have told many of you— things happen for a reason and I want to say that I am very happy to have her here during this particular time. She's been a big help and it's nice to have her company.

We have the best of both worlds, because she has many weekend horse shows, so we are not constantly in each other's faces, which could probably get old fast. So, for the next few months, I think this is going to work out fine and then I expect that another Divine Intervention will take her to the next place that she should be.

So-o-o, until the next time, I want to thank you for your continued prayers and good wishes, the cards, the phone calls, the dinners, the soup, the ginger snaps, the haircut, the house cleaning, and the emails.
I love you guys!!!! Carla

Trish sent a few ideas for the top ten list:
- Say goodbye to bad hair days.
- Ride on the back of his motorcycle without worrying about the wind-blown hairdo.
- If you are short on money, you can work at Taco Bell without a hairnet.
- Make all your girlfriend's envious by getting ready in 10 minutes!
- Hot and humid weather? Not to worry! This head is cool!
- Be a real trend-setter. Don't forget the BIG earrings!

Patty sent a few good things that she experienced while going through chemo:
- We learn that life without alcohol is pretty darn entertaining.
- We attract men like a magnet— it seems they like to see the soft side of a strong woman (and our soft side does surface, doesn't it?)
- We QUIT worrying about the small stuff.
- When we order a half a sandwich, they bring us a whole— plus a cookie—and an extra loaf of bread to take home (they want us to gain weight).
- We can arrive LATE and leave EARLY without guilt.
- We start talking to more people...just because we can.
- We slow down long enough to really hear what people are saying—then life begins to feel surreal, because there is so much clarity.

And a last reason from Maureen who was going through her own "cancer" experience via her new job:

> Carla~ I know another reason for your having chemo, however, it may not be top 10 material, but here goes..."so you can teach your neophyte-rookie breast cancer nurse friend how to help breast cancer patients through their experience."

I once read that if you ever wondered how you would "handle" losing a loved one through death, that you should look back on past situations in your life during which you experienced grief (loss of a marriage, loss of a job, etc.) and it would give you a picture of how you would handle the grief process through any future losses.

This may also summarize how one might expect to handle living through chemotherapy.

I decided that my approach to chemotherapy was going to be much like any other life challenge that I had experienced in the past—just face it head on...learn as much about it as possible...take it one day at a time, but continue through it with a strong "I can do it" attitude.

For me, this was like a boxing match that I was going to win! That being said, there were times when I realized that sometimes I was winning the fight and other times I was fighting to win. With each successive treatment, I felt like I was knocked down to the mat. I had eight treatments scheduled...and after each one, I realized that I was closer to being finished with this fight. So, every time, I struggled to get back up on my feet and was ready—yes, even looking forward to—the next round.

> Date: Wednesday, March 17, 2004
> To: My Prayer Group
> Subject: Metamorphosis-Part IX: Chemo Countdown 3
> *Happy moments, praise God. Difficult moments, seek God. Quiet moments, worship God. Painful moments, trust God. Every moment, thank God.*—Author Unknown
>
> OK...To those of you who have said I have been an inspiration, I confess—I am a whiner, weenie, wuss. I would rather have 8 surgeries than these chemo treatments!!
>
> From the very beginning, I told my doctor that I have a high tolerance for pain and a low tolerance for drugs. It seems that I know myself pretty well, because it takes me about 7 days to recuperate from a treatment. I probably have whined to most of

you by now and I am making no bones about the fact that chemo sucks!!!...and I hope NONE of you ever have to go through it.

That being said, I have one more of the Adriamycin and Cytoxan combo (it makes me nauseated just to write those words) and then four of the Taxotere. I am completely bald, although I still have eyebrows, eyelashes and have to shave my legs (go figure?)

Nadine graciously accompanied me to my last treatment and, even though I complain, I continue to count my blessings for the number of true friends that are in my life.

Marge came over on Saturday to plant some beautiful flowers on my back patio and then stayed with me because I was not feeling so hot. I have to admit that even in my queasy state, I was worried about HER—especially when she kept talking to the plants, telling them that they have a new home and they should stay pretty for her friend, Carla. WOW!! I have heard about people talking to their plants...but I didn't know they REALLY did that!!! I want you to know that I put in the plant food today, as instructed...but I really felt STOOOPID talking to the plants. I don't know how long they will survive—which is why I have silk plants throughout my house!

I have a big weekend planned...this is the weekend of the Winter Park Art Show—which means great art and fabulous jazz in the park. It is also the Bay Hill Golf Tournament weekend—which means a party at Sandy and Van's—who live near the 17th hole. We walk around looking for Tiger Woods. No—I really don't care about golf, but it is a time to "see and be seen"!!! I don't know if I will wear my long wig, my short wig or a colorful scarf with a BIG hat! Oh, so many choices. I am just thankful that this is an "off" week for the chemo.

I continue to thank God for each and every one of you in my life and hope that—if I don't see you anytime soon that, at least, we will talk—if not, know that you are in my prayers, as I hope I am in yours.

Love to all, Carla

Carla,

You *are* in my thoughts and prayers. Chemo sucks—especially Adriamycin!! Taxotere should be better. Love, Patty

Hey Carla,

You are no whiney, weenie person. You are entitled to some anger, annoyance and all the other feelings you have. But praise God you are on the downside of chemo. Of course the 7th day is the downside, because that is when the drugs actually kick in. I pray for you every day, and know that this time next year; you will be looking back at a period that only made you stronger. Love ya, Maur

Good Luck Carla.

It sounds like you are remaining as positive as can be. I'd go with the long wig...You look hot in it! Have a good time this weekend. Justin, your favorite godson.

CJ-

I spent quite a bit of time yesterday with an old business acquaintance who was diagnosed with leukemia last year. He is about 50 years old. He went through all the chemo and is currently in remission, has regrown hair, and is able to work a pretty full schedule. I temporarily put aside my selfish side and spent several hours with him.

Told him a little about your situation.

Prayers for you. BRW

Sent: Mar 30, 2004 6:00 PM
To: My Prayer Group
Subject: Metamorphosis – Part X: Halfway there
Our cells are constantly eavesdropping on our thoughts and being changed by them. A bout of depression can wreak havoc with the immune system; falling in love can boost it. Despair and helplessness raise the risk of heart attacks and cancer, thereby shortening life. Joy and fulfillment keep us healthy and extend life. This means that the line between biology and psychology can't really be drawn with any certainty. A remembered stress, which is only a wisp of thought, releases the same flood of destructive hormones as the stress itself.
—Deepak Chopra

My long-time friend and nursing school roomie, Maureen, sent me the quote above...take heed. Hm-m-m-m. It looks like I need to fall in love. However, I do love all of you and I hope that counts, because it certainly boosts my system when I think of each of you and how loving and supportive you have all been, particularly over these past several months. I am half-way through treatment and the Adriamycin/Cytoxan combo is finished—Halleluiah!!!! My friend, Linda, agreed to accompany me on this treatment and had her husband, Alan, pick me up prior to my meeting her at the Cancer Center.

This week, I had an unusually "energetic" exchange with Dr. Gorgeous and his nurse practitioner. I don't know why, but Dr. G. asked me if the lunch I had today involved a "keg" and Linda said I was "wired". Only God knows when those energetic moments come—or go. Thank you, Linda and Alan again for taking the time out of your life to accompany me to the doc and chemo today and for the chicken soup.

I don't know how one can possibly enjoy the chemo experience; but I must say that it was enjoyable??? I believe it has to do with the trust and the humor and the love that surrounds me and those who are in my world.

With the new medicine for nausea that I took this time: (for those who are interested: Emend: 3 pills=$308.00—Yes, that was also a topic I discussed with the doc), No...I was not nauseated, but how would I know, since I slept for 3 days straight????!!!

My hemoglobin is down to 10.6 (from 12.6) and I am feeling that my energy is zapped. I look like the Procrit commercials where gramps can't go upstairs to get his camera to take pictures of the kids, because he has no energy. I CAN RELATE! Hopefully, the hemoglobin will be below 10 next time, so I can get a shot of that stuff. (Dr. G. only gives the Procrit if the hemoglobin goes below 10).

Today, I went to lunch at the Olive Garden with Beth (my co-worker and friend from Priority). I ordered everything on the menu! Steak Gorgonzola with pasta, salad, and breadsticks with Alfredo sauce (load me up on calories!!!). I only ate half and took the rest home. Thank you, Beth, not only for meeting me for lunch, but for paying for my meal, which will last me for the next week!!

I have to admit though; I didn't feel well after the meal. I don't know if it was too heavy (ya think?) or it was the energy thing, but by the time I got home, I threw off my wig and called Linda's husband, Alan, who has time and again offered to do some "healing energy" work on me.

This man has a gift—after an hour of energy work, he cleared something in me that was "bogging me down". He also touched on some type of "joyful spirit" in me, because as he was finishing, he started to chuckle and couldn't stop! I am grateful to you, Alan, because I truly feel lighter and feel my energy flowing again. In fact, after he left, I vacuumed the whole downstairs (which I personally haven't done for weeks—but, don't tell Kelly!)

This weekend, I hope to be dancing at Trish's birthday party; and next weekend, my favorite Easter Bunnie is coming to town—my sister, Jan Jan, (whose alias is Bunnie Ghirardelli)...and lucky her, she gets to accompany me to my next treatment!!!

So, as always, I have many things to look forward to—please keep me in your prayers as you are all in mine.

Til the next time...Love and light to all...

Carla (aka Mimi Godiva)

11. Creating Joyful Moments

'Today you can make your life significant and worthwhile. The present is yours to do with as you will.'
—Grenville Kleiser, American Writer

When you are on the outside looking in at a breast cancer patient's life, I am sure it is difficult to fathom how joyful life can be for her. I am here to tell you that some of my most enjoyable moments took place on the day of my chemotherapy treatments.

Date: 4-16-2004
To: My Prayer Group
Subject: Metamorphosis - Part XI
'Life isn't about finding yourself. Life is about creating yourself.'
—George Bernard Shaw

Well...I really didn't think I would make it this far (after my 2nd chemo treatment, I called my mom and told her I was going to quit the treatments)...but, as of today—I am "over the hump".

I started the second half of treatment with the first round of Taxol last Friday...so I have three Taxol treatments to go. I found it to be rather coincidental that I started the Adriamycin/Cytoxan on Friday the 13th and started my Taxol on Good Friday. (Hm-m-m??)

Anyway, my sister, Janis flew in from Chicago to be with Kelly and me on Easter. Since Friday was a holiday for me (first place I ever worked where Good Friday is a holiday!), I picked her up at the airport and I spied her immediately, since she was walking toward me with her bunny ears on!!

We went directly to the Cancer Center to have my treatment (some vacation, huh?). BUT, not before we had a little "Bunnie (Janis's alter ego) and Mimi (MY alter ego) experience".

I guess I need to preface the actual "Bunnie and Mimi experience" with a little background info—first, I must admit that I have lost about 6 pounds since my surgery/chemo—which I can't afford. And as you know, I have not been getting to the gym as often as I would like (due to recovery/nausea) so needless to say, I have pretty much *lost my bootie.*

Last week, as I was trying on a size 6 pantsuit, I mentioned to the sales lady that I no longer have a butt! She told me that she used to work at Frederick's of Hollywood where one could "buy a butt for $27.00!"

I said: "Really?? You're serious???...I want one!!!"

So, I went to the mall...walked straight into Frederick's of Hollywood and said: "I need to buy a butt!" Sure enough, the saleslady pulled one out and the price tag was $27.00.

"Do you want a black or white butt?" the saleslady asked.

"A WHITE butt, of course!" I said, *What is she thinking?* "Let me try a medium and a small".

I took my jeans off, put on the medium butt, tore off the price tag, put my jeans back on and paid for the butt. I am telling you—I looked BETTER than J-Lo!!!

Suddenly, when I was about halfway home, it dawned on me that when the saleswoman at Frederick's asked me if I wanted a black butt or white butt...she was really asking me if I wanted the *panty* in black or white.

Now...I don't own any white panties...so I was really upset that I just spent $27.00 on a white butt, when I really WANTED a BLACK butt. OMG...I think "chemo brain" has set in!!!

Okay, back to my story...

After I picked up JanJan (aka "Bunnie"), we stopped for a bite to eat before chemo. As we were eating, we cracked up as I told her my Frederick's butt story. As we were walking out of Boston Market, we were looking in the large picture window, comparing butts—and, much to our surprise, WE WERE CAUGHT—by an African American man in a van, passing by, who shouted: "LOOKING GOOD!!!" So, I guess it doesn't matter if my butt is black or white! Huh?!!!

So-o-o, we get to the Dr. Molthrop's office (Janis calls it "The Chemo Place") and I am wearing the bunny ears (over my short wig) and we go in and start telling Sally and Kathy (the girls at the front desk) our butt story (I tell them EVERYTHING!). A patient is standing there as I say: "Yes, I have fake hair, fake boobs and now a fake butt!"

She was surprised and asked: "Is that a WIG? It looks GREAT!! (Everyone says that who finds out it's not my hair.)

Well, ole' Bunnie pipes up: "Everything I HAVE is REAL!" (AS IF it's all about HER??? Duh!!)

And the patient says: "Really? I thought YOU were wearing a wig!!" HA-ha-ha-ha-ha-haaaaa!!!!

Needless to say...another FUN trip to "The Chemo Place".

Post chemo, this time was pretty uneventful...no nausea or queasiness. In fact, on Saturday, we went to the Chihuly Exhibit at the Art Museum; and on Sunday, Janis made a great Easter dinner (and I helped). She even cleaned up the house (while I napped) before our friends arrived.

We had 8 people for Easter dinner, including Kelly, Trish and her son, Richard; Marge and Ed Brennan and Ed's 90-year old mother, Margaret—who I was most honored to have, because she generally only goes out of the house for doctor's appointments.

Over the course of the afternoon, Janis drank a whole bottle of wine and was quite entertaining (actually, no one could get a word in edgewise!) and although I had no wine, I had two helpings of everything...which was quite extraordinary.

The weekend was great...I really enjoyed having my sister down, so that she could see that I am looking GOOD and feeling fine. And sharing Easter with friends and family was joyous!

I forgot to tell you that on Saturday, Janis also took a number of pictures of me (so that I can remember the experience of being bald...and other body re-designs). We got a little crazy...both she and Kelly used lipstick to write and draw on a number of my body parts. It truly was a memorable day! Jan Jan has mailed me a CD of all of the photos, which one day, I will share with each of you (well, MOST of you). I am attaching a couple with this email; but the more risqué ones, I will save for my "Post Chemo Celebration Party", which I am beginning to plan...to celebrate YOU, my family and my friends!

Well, I am sure that you have had enough of this memoir...but know that I love you all; you are in my heart and I pray daily for your good health and happiness.

The joy of living is so precious and I am more "in tune" each day. Divine interventions continue as I share my story with the right people at the right time. I am amazed by all of this. I am also amazed and grateful to the number of people who are praying for me...many of them whom I will never know...but will be blessed for their caring thoughts and prayers.

Til the next time...

In light and love,

Carla/Mimi

Car-

You are confirmation that bald is beautiful! What beautiful features you have. I LOVE the photo showing just the back of your head—who wrote "Mimi" on your head with lipstick??? Are you guys crazy???

...And, by the way, the one with you in the wig, is very chic. I want to borrow it when you no longer need it.

Love Maur

Mimi —

I sent this photo to my pals, to let them know how fabulous you look. They all responded in agreement. Below is Blake's response. He is so-o-o Blake! Love, JanJan

> Janis,
> Thanks for the photo. Carla looks amazing! I'm so glad you had the opportunity to spend some time with her. Tell her that I recommend she wear that hairstyle when her hair comes back. WOW! She looks absolutely gorgeous. Please tell her I said so.
> Love you, Blake

Hey Lalalalalalala,

Glad you are hanging in there!!! It sounds like The Easter Bunny was good to you. The photos didn't come through to my computer. Try it again and send some of the censored ones, which I am sure, are the good ones!! Take care of yourself and know that you are in my thoughts and prayers every day!!!
xxoo helen

> Helen~
> OH NO!!...I am not sending the censored ones...I may one day see myself on the internet with some weird saying underneath—Like:
> Bilateral Mastectomies - $50,000
> A bald head from chemo - $15,000
> A butt from Frederick's of Hollywood - $27.00
> This X-rated picture: Priceless!
> ~Carla

Carla-

It was good to hear from you. You're looking great!!!! I know that you will be happy when chemo is over. I think about and pray for you regularly.

I am going for a run in a while and will meditate with you in mind—while dodging old women.

I think I might enjoy seeing some of the other pictures.........
BRW

Car~

All I can say is God Bless and I love you. Your humor is so divine, but I always knew that. I think one of our earliest divine interventions was being roomies in nursing school ~Maur

Yes Maur...that is the truth...

I didn't even know what "divine intervention" meant when we were roomies—but God certainly did place you in my life. Yesterday, I was thinking about the numerous people who have crossed my path in this life and am grateful for the very "special ones" who have remained in my life years after we were physically apart. You don't know how blessed I feel, because I have so many of these wonderful soul mates in my life and they, like you, are standing by me...closer than ever. I love you dearly Maur...Car

Hi Carla,

Just want to say 'hey' and tell you that I am so glad you had so much fun with your sister...nothing better than a sister who is a friend...sounds like you had a great time with her!!! Loved both of the butt stories!

I went to Raleigh to spend Easter with my friend Beth and her family. She has two great teenage boys and they love it in NC.

You are in my prayers...isn't it amazing—the power of prayer? I admire your attitude and coping skills. I know that you feel the security of God's love.
Olga

Hey Sweetie~

The pictures are great! And the butt story is hilarious—it was so-o-o-o you! I'm glad you're finished with the "red devil", and are having an easier time with the Taxol. You're almost done, and very much alive & kicking—and that's what matters.

Keep your stories coming—they always give me a lift. Can't wait to see you.
Love, Prissy

My Dear Carla,

You are such a bright light. Your spirit warms me and your strength is amazing. On top of that, you look great! You don't look like you aged a day since I saw you last fall. I wish I could be with you and spend time catching up but for now we must communicate by email. I miss you and love you.

May God continue to bless you with all his choice Blessings.
Love, Pat S.

Aunt Carla~

Thanks for the email! I'm glad to hear that you are almost finished with the chemo! You looked great in the pics! I thought I would send you this...Love, Erin

> *This morning when I wakened,*
> *And saw the sun above,*
> *I softly said, "Good morning, Lord,*
> *Bless everyone I love."*
>
> *And, right away I thought of you,*
> *And said a loving prayer,*
> *That He would bless you specially,*
> *And keep you free from care.*
> *I thought of all the happiness*
> *A day could hold in store.*
> *I wished it all for you because*
> *No one deserves it more.*

12. Having Faithful Friends and Family

'Under pressure, your faith-life is forced into the open and shows its true colors.' —James, Jesus' Disciple

The saying goes that "you find out who your true friends really are when you go through some type of trouble or need". Living through the ordeal of a breast cancer diagnosis—and all that it entails—certainly puts that statement to the test.

I have always thought that my family and friends were not only loving and giving, but loyal to me as a person. However, not everyone has an opportunity to go through life...and actually have confirmation that these faithful relationships are real and lasting.

Throughout this experience, my family and friends have proven over and over again that their relationships with me are real...and I am blessed to have them in my life.

Date: April 30, 2004
To: My Prayer Group
Subject: Metamorphosis - Part XII
'We are pressed on every side by troubles, but we are not crushed and broken. We are perplexed, but we don't give up and quit. We are hunted down, but God never abandons us. We get knocked down, but we get up again and keep going'—Paul: 2 Corinthians 4:8-9.

Hello Everyone! Six treatments done and two to go...

This past week my friend Sue came to my rescue, by giving up almost a full work day to take me to my second Taxol treatment. Sue has "come through in a clutch" for me several times throughout this ordeal—during my surgery, post-op and driving me to the plastic surgeon's office for my drain removal—and has had the opportunity to observe my attempts at "advocating" for myself with the healthcare professionals. So, she was probably prepared for the interactions that I seem to enjoy when I go to "The Chemo Place".

We arrived at Dr. Molthrop's office at 11:30am and after a few minutes of harassing the front desk staff; I went in to get weighed. I am happy to report that I gained a pound!!!

The medical assistants, as always, were perplexed by my joy at this news. But, when I told them I was on a "weight gain" diet, they started with the flip-flop hand rub to "transfer their pounds" to me. One of the bigger and beautiful medical assistants even turned me around and we rubbed butts, so that her pounds could rub onto mine. (DON'T WORRY; this is not another butt story!)

After I had my blood drawn, Sue and I were escorted into the exam room to meet with Dr. Molthrop aka Dr. Gorgeous.

When Dr. G. came in, I introduced Sue. He mentioned that I "always bring a different friend with me" when I visit him and he proceeded to ask Sue how much I *paid* her to come...because he "KNOWS I can't have that many friends!" (YUK-yuk...Dr. "Straight Laced" Molthrop is FINALLY starting to develop a sense of humor!!)

After we all had a little chuckle at *my expense*, I started firing off my questions—along with telling both Dr. G. and the nurse practitioner about some of the side effects that I had been experiencing.

"I am having fatigue", I emphasized the point by saying, "You've seen the commercials—I need some Procrit!"

"Well, your hemoglobin is up one tenth of a point this week" he said almost gleefully, "and we only give Procrit if it goes below 10". *Damn!*

Then I start talking about the glutamine that I have to take to diminish the potential for neuropathy (nerve damage) and said that I had to shell out $70 for it at the health food store (not covered by insurance). But, I tell him that I want to sell it to his patients and asked if he would let me do that. He agreed to it and I say: "Of course, you can't get a "kickback" because it's against the Stark laws (it's illegal)". In exasperation, he says: "You have everything covered, don't you?" (You have got to know that Dr. G. LOVES me.)

Fifteen minutes later, he starts to leave and I said: "Hey, what about my hug? My friend, Barbara, who is also your patient, says that you ALWAYS give her a hug when you leave the room."

He said: "You intimidate me!" But, he came back and gave me a hug.

Huh? I intimidate HIM? I suppose my "spirit" is stronger than ever...and that's a good thing.

Anyway, last weekend, following chemo, I felt like I was going to faint every time I stood up—uhhhh-hello...LOW hemoglobin!!! So, I had to cancel plans to see "The Red Coats" (a Dave Clark Five/Beatles-type band) with a bunch of friends. I am dying to get out and have some fun!

This weekend all my friends are gone, so I don't know what I am going to do with myself. Maybe I will go shopping. I need to buy some new clothes since I still haven't gained back all of my pre-chemo weight.

I have been laying low this week—I worked three days with my boss, Nathan, who came up from Miami. After having done that, I must say, I am in the right job at the right time. This man is the most enthusiastic, caring man I have ever met in my 30-some years of work. He is so supportive and complimentary, that I just can't believe it. He said I was "one tough lady", because he hasn't seen any decline in my performance throughout the treatment period. And, when I told him I only have two treatments left, he stated: "It really went fast!" (It truly must seem that way to those who aren't actually experiencing this ordeal!)

Otherwise, this week has been uneventful...I continue to read "The Purpose Driven Life", which has opened my eyes about why we are all challenged during our lifetime...and that God never said that we only get challenged once. God uses problems to draw us closer to Himself. These challenges are just incidents in God's plan for us. I truly believe that—and that belief is probably what has carried me through these past several months...along with all of your support, of course.

One thing Nathan said to me this week, which I thought was quite profound..."Soon you'll be back to your old self—but you will be different."...and he is right—the two are not mutually exclusive...and I look forward to my "new life"—my Metamorphosis.

So, until the next time, I thank you for your prayers for my continued healing...you are all in my prayers each day as I thank God for what and whom I have in my life.
In love and light,
Carla

Chesser,
Thanks for the ongoing updates on your progress. No, I have to agree, you will never be your old self again, nor would you ever want to be.

I'm glad to hear you got a hug out of Molthrop. He is a pretty shy guy, and I guess because I am so short, I don't intimidate him, which is why he hugs me!! Ha!

I am also reading The Purpose Driven Life—I'm on day 21. My priest friend was reading the book and he recommended the book to me. My only criticism is that I can't read just one chapter a night. I have this tendency to want to read ahead.

Yes, we missed you last Saturday night at Dexter's. We had quite a table full of people and The Red Coats were great, as always. How about Dexter's tomorrow night? Are you up to it?
Barbara

Carla~

Thank God things are going so well for you, I guess our prayers are really getting up to Him. I don't know if you have ever heard this poem but I dig it out often and reflect on it:

My life is but a weaving between my God and
me. I do not choose the colors; He worketh
steadily.
Oftimes He weaveth sorrow, and I in foolish
pride, forget He sees both upper and under side.
Not til the loom is silent and shuttle cease to fly,
Will God unroll the canvas and explain the
reason WHY.
The dark threads are as needful in the skillful
weaver's hand
As the threads of gold and silver in the pattern
He has planned.
                                    Love, Mom and Dad

Carla,

Your stories sound oh so familiar, but are somewhat different. My oncologist is female! I go in for an MRI mid-May...and am looking forward to having that over with. I am feeling a bit melancholy this week...not really LOW per se, just reflective on the whole ordeal.
You are in my thoughts, Much Love, Patty

Dear Carla,

Jo here...I am sitting in the Crown Room in New Orleans and am on my way home. So glad to hear that you are through six of the treatments already. I am so sorry we were unable to come through for you last week...I wasn't home and Craig had 3 appointments himself that day. I figured if we got a second e-mail from you asking for help that he would change them. What an ordeal and how much you are learning! It is truly amazing.

I will let you know as soon as I see some brief light in the schedule so we can get together for lunch. Right now it is

looking like it might be awhile. But you are first on my list. Stay
well dear friend.
Love, Jo (and Craig)

Hi Carla,

Alan and I are in Europe on vacation! We're having an
incredible time. Will tell you about it when I come back next
Friday. I wanted you to know that we went to Notre Dame in
Paris and I lit a candle for you and my children's great uncle,
Sonny, who started chemo last week. I hope you felt the spirit.

Talk to you soon. Thanks for the window into your
incredible journey. Love, Linda

Oh, Carla! This is the best one ever!

I love what you said about the future. No surprise that you
intimidate Dr. Gorgeous. You can bet he's blessed by you and
your incredible spirit!

I tried to reach you today...wondering where you are THIS
week. I'm so glad you have Nathan. What an insightful guy and
great boss! You are truly blessed to be with that company and
made the absolutely right choice. It's serendipitous how things
turned out. I so look forward to the end of your treatment...it's
just around the corner.

I continue to be amazed and inspired by you, dear one.
I love you,
Trish

Dear Carla,

Been thinking of you a lot.....

I have saved all your 'metamorphosis' essays—they are
wonderful commentary and worthy of publishing if you ever
decide to seek a wider audience for your very unique
perspective on a journey too many women have to make. I
know, unfortunately, that there will be more friends/family
afflicted (even me, possibly) down the road; I will have your
words to offer to these others as a special gift of spiritual
hangin' on and encouragement...and laughter!
Love you...
Beth

As I said, my faithful friends are not only faithful to me, but
have a lot of faith in the Source of our Divine Inspiration. *How
Blessed can one person be?*

13. Seeing the Light

O Beautiful Affliction; Merciful pain
This mortal wounding bringing me to life again
In suffering there's healing
This darkness revealing
Silence speaking volumes to my soul
O Beautiful Affliction
Blessed brokenness that makes me whole

—David Baroni

Date: Friday, May 7, 2004
To: My Prayer Group
Subject: Metamorphosis - Part XIII
'You never know how brave you can be, until you are called upon to be brave.'—Author Unknown
This quote was given to me by a friend at the gym, whose sister carried the quote around in her pocket before she died of breast cancer...soon after I was diagnosed.

Section A: *(This section is being written under the influence of Benadryl...having JUST come from chemo, I am still a little LOOPY!)*

Dear Friends and Family: The cocoon is starting to open...and the butterfly is ready to soar'—only ONE more treatment to go!!!

This week, Kelly's friend, Michelle was gracious enough to "pinch hit" and accompany me to chemo when Kay had to cancel due to unforeseen work obligations. *Can you imagine?!!* Anyway, I think Michelle was a little nervous, so I prepared her for exactly what was going to take place.

I wore a pair of capris—which were a little big, so I had to wear my "butt" this time and, of course, everyone in the office had heard about my "Frederick's of Hollywood butt", so they all asked if I had it on. As you can imagine, I was *shakin' booty* and showing it off all day long.

We went in to see Dr. Molthrop and I introduced Michelle by saying: "This is my daughter's best friend...I have used up all of my friends, so now I am working on my daughter's friends". He looked at sweet, young Michelle...and bit his tongue.

The visit was uneventful; questions, questions, smart-ass remarks, questions, interruptions, more questions and more smart-ass remarks. Same ole', same ole.

131

However, when Dr. G. was ready to leave (after he helped me up to a sitting position on the treatment table), HE asked ME for a hug, so I stood on the step of the treatment table—which put me up at about 7'0, so I leaned over to him at 6'3" and said: "See now I AM taller than you!"

Of course, we had to re-hash the "you intimidate me" story and I told him that I wrote about him in my emails.

He said: "You don't really intimidate me...you..."

"Harrass you", I interrupted.

"No...you are..."

"Pushy", I interrupted a second time.

"NO...you are doing it now!" He was just barely aggravated.

"I finish your sentences?" I quipped.

"Yes, you do that...but, what I want to say is that you are the type of patient who takes charge of their care...and challenges...and asks questions...and THAT's a good thing...I like patients like that. You are..."

"PRICKLY", I said.

"YES!!!!!" he agreed.

So, how do you like that? My doctor is intimidated by me AND he thinks I am prickly.

I told him he was too straight and needed to lighten up. Then, he went into a 5 minute dissertation as to why he has to be "professional and serious" until he gets to know someone and determines their emotional state...blah-blah-blah. ANOTHER FUN DAY WITH DR. G.!!! (I have to be careful...or he may order another round of treatments.)

Next, we went into the treatment room, where they call me "Bob Hope" Chesser and my primary job is to "entertain the troops". I actually think I am "channeling" Bob Hope, because I get going and just can't stop!

At one point, Michelle walked me to the bathroom (she pushed the IV pole because I was loopy from the Benadryl) and when I came out, I yelled: "Who left the seat up? I fell into the toilet!!!" (A man had gone in before me—so I pointed at him when I came out). The place was roaring with laughter!! (They're gonna miss me when I am gone).

I ate the whole time I was there (it was most likely from the steroid, Decadron)...ginger cookies and a Zone Bar—I even got food from one of the other patients. Her son, Chad (FSU Football team fullback or maybe it's linebacker—anyway, he wears #45 on the field) had gone out to get some food from Wendy's and was carrying a couple of bags back into the treatment room. So, of course, I gave him a hard time about not asking ME if I wanted to order something. He asked: "Do you want a salad?" (Apparently he had bought three for himself—he's HUGE!!!).

I said: "No, I want the chicken nuggets"...and GUESS WHAT HE PULLED OUT OF THE BAG? YES, CHICKEN NUGGETS (Not only am I channeling Bob, but I have ESP!) So, he brings over the box...and of course, I had to take one.

Then the front office girls, Sally and Kathy, came back and I asked when were they popping popcorn (remember when I was taking the Adriamycin/Cytoxan—the odor of the popcorn made me sick??!!). At 3:00pm, they brought me half a bag of popcorn!!! And, it was DELISH!!

One of the other ladies receiving chemo, Cheryl, is on the same treatment regime that I am—and May 20th is her last treatment also, so we spent an hour planning our "HALLELUIAH'—WE'RE FINISHED" party. I am taking balloons and an entrée (Egg salad—with NO relish) and she is bringing Mocha Cheesecake (She works at Ruth's Chris Steakhouse). Of course, I have to bring something in for the nurses—LOTS AND LOTS OF SUGAR!!!

Oh...something interesting—last Friday, April 30th, my friend, Diana did an "all night-er" Relay for Life—Breast Cancer fundraiser (it was a horrible weather day—rain, lightning, thunder, so I didn't go)...and she called me at 9:30pm and said: "I was walking around the lake and I had 3 luminaries lit"—"one for Jackie", a friend of hers who died of breast cancer a few years ago—"one for my aunt" who also was being treated for cancer and—"one for you".

She said: "The only one that is still lit is YOURS!" I got goose bumps and said: "That's because my light is shining bright inside me!" She screamed excitedly: "I know! It's D.I.!!" (Divine Intervention—Diana is now a believer).

The sad thing is that Diana's aunt died the next day. So, she is in my prayers.

Okay...it's 6:15pm, and I am getting hungry...so, I will finish this at a later date---when I am not so loopy and not so hungry.

Section B: (Writing this on Friday after a conversation with my sister Jan Jan—aka Bunnie)

I am feeling good so far today, a day after chemo...hoping it will last through the weekend because I have a 50th birthday party for my friend, Gay, tomorrow evening and...of course, Sunday is Mother's Day and I was invited to Marge's house to celebrate with her family. Her two sons from New York, Justin (my god-ness son) and Christian and his two children are down for the weekend.

Anyway, another interesting occurrence happened today—something we shall continue to call "D.I."

My sister, Janis, was in her office talking on the phone to her friend this afternoon. Apparently, the day in Chicago was dreary and cloudy; however, while on the phone, Janis looked out and the sky was clearing and the sun started shining. All of a sudden she sees a yellow Monarch butterfly outside her office window!!

She mentioned this to her friend, and said: "I believe that is Carla—her symbol is the butterfly!" And her friend said: "Hang up and call her"....and so, she did. But, I didn't answer the phone (because I was "flying outside her window, of course.) Actually, I was at the doctor's office getting my LAST shot of Neulasta (to increase my White Blood Cell count—this has been my routine all along, but I may not have mentioned it—as opposed to Procrit, which is given to increase the Red Blood Cell count—and which I never received).

On the way home, I went to use my cell phone and picked up Janis' message about the butterfly...and was thinking about the symbolism and how blessed I have been throughout this process.

Just then I noticed the car in front of me and smiled as I read its license plate: "WE COVRU". Then I looked at the car to its right, which had a license plate that read: "MERCY 4U"....and I knew I was getting a divine message! Isn't that awesome????

Janis just called again and we discussed the butterfly...and she said not only was she astonished that she had seen the butterfly—but was amazed that it was outside her 5th floor window!!! She said that "I brought the Florida sunshine with me (aka the butterfly)...and when the butterfly left—the dreariness returned...then, when she told her friend that "I didn't answer the phone, she said: "Of course she didn't...she was up here!" Amazing, huh?!!

Well, I think I am going to send this out today, because it is a little long and I have another two weeks before my LAST, yes, my LAST treatment!

So, if anything significant happens, I will send another email before my LAST treatment. In the meantime, I will keep you all in my prayers and hope that each of you are aware of the D.I. in your life, as they occur EVERYDAY.

Bless you all and thank you for your continued prayers. Happy Mother's Day to all of you moms out there and keep an eye out for the butterflies!
In love and light,
Carla

Carla,
Loved your message...the stories about The Chemo Place are hilarious! You really could write a book. I have a few similar stories...and I notice D.I. via my dogs. They help me every single day. I sing to them in the morning; I imitate them at work all day and I get down on the floor and play with them in the evening. They keep things light, and keep me moving.
They were actually born the week I had my lumpectomy. They were 8 weeks old when I got them. They have brought so much joy and purpose to my life. They help me keep things in perspective.
Have a fabulous weekend! You are in my thoughts.
Patty

Carla~
Great message...they ARE going to miss you at Dr.G's office when this is all over! Your big heart shows in the way that you care, Carla.
God knows our hearts...I just know He is smiling on you and about you!!! Olga

CJ—
Perhaps you are channeling Colonel Sanders?????
BRW

Love it. Love it. Love you. Trish

Date: Saturday, May 8th
Subject: Thank you, Sweetie
Michelle~
I wanted to tell you how much I appreciate your taking the day yesterday to escort me to my treatment. You were a lifesaver! I am grateful to have had you share the experience with me and hope I didn't embarrass you throughout the process! You are a wonderful "daughter" and a very special friend to Kelly. Thank you for being there for both of us.
I love you!
Carla (Your second Mom)

14. The Butterfly Emerges

'Never consent to creep when you feel compelled to soar'

—Helen Keller

Date: May 27, 2004
To: My Prayer Group
Subject: Metamorphosis - Part XIV: Last Treatment
'Life is a test...Life is a trust'—The Purpose-Driven Life

HIP HIP HOORAY! The chemo treatment is over...and the butterfly is starting to emerge!

Sorry, I haven't written sooner, but Priscilla (from California) took some time to come visit me this weekend and we were on the go the entire weekend...on Friday, we went to dinner and then saw the most hilarious musical "Menopause—The Musical". On Saturday, we went shopping for about 4 hours and then went to a "Rhapsody in the Springs" philharmonic concert under the stars; and on Sunday we had a fabulous dinner with Marge.

Priscilla and I spent a lot of time on my "lanai" (as she called it) and each time we sat out there, we saw one or two Monarch butterflies...in fact, I have been seeing them a lot lately—a message that I believe is meant for me.

...so, I hope those are good enough reasons for not writing until now.

Plus, I have been working...and going to the gym...and I had a date on Tuesday night (don't get excited) and then, of course I had to watch American Idol last night....so-o-o...

...I will go all the way back to May 20th and share with you my last treatment "scenario"...

Originally, Marge offered to take me to my last treatment (she was the one who accompanied me in November to my first meeting with my oncologist, Dr. Gorgeous.) Kelly also mentioned that she wanted to take me to my last treatment, hoping that she wouldn't have to be away for a horse show. So, it was obvious to me that—not only did I have a plan, but I had a *back-up plan* (what have we learned about CONTROL over these past six months???)

Well, my plan AND my back-up plan actually *back-fired!!* Marge called me to let me know that she had to travel to Rochester for a meeting, so she couldn't take me—so I said: "That's ok, Kelly can take me"...but when I asked Kelly, she—

thinking that Marge was taking me—had scheduled two new clients for riding lessons in West Palm Beach AND she had a horse show! So, I was up the proverbial creek...

What to do?? I couldn't think of anyone who would be available to take me to my treatment, which started at 9:45 am. I knew that I could drive myself to The Cancer Center, but it was the driving home (under the influence of Benadryl) that I wasn't too sure about. So, I figured well, I could just hang around until the Benadryl "loopy-ness" wore off and then I would be able to drive. So, in my mind, I was prepared to do that.

As it happened, I went to the gym on the Tuesday night before my Thursday treatment and shared my dilemma with Nadine. Nadine immediately said: "NO...we will find someone to take you:" And, not five minutes later, she came over to me and said that her daughter, Jessica, would take me to the treatment; and our friend at the gym, Terri, would pick me up and take me home. Problem solved (we will have to call this one N.I.—Nadine Intervention!!) Thanks to all of you!

The night before chemo day, I went to the grocery store to buy something for the staff at Dr. G's office. First, I had a variety of *desserts* in the shopping cart—but thought, no—and I took them out. Then, I put in a *bunch of fruit* (which I would have to cut and arrange on a tray)—too much work—I took them out. I then searched and searched and finally found the PERFECT food...something that was memorable to all of us— POPCORN!!! Yes, the smell of which caused me to be nauseous every time I went into the office for my first four treatments and the very same thing that on my 7th treatment, I couldn't scarf down fast enough. I bought them SIX boxes of various types!!!

Next, I got home and tried to figure out what to wear for my last treatment. I put on the leopard print scarf (that my sister, Bunnie had given me) and my big floppy black beach hat—Yes! I thought...THIS and a pair of big black sunglasses would be perfect!

On Thursday morning, Jessica dropped me off at The Cancer Center and I walked into the office at 9:45am with my goodie bag in hand—I had chickened out with the hat and sunglasses— but WISH I had worn them—it would have been SUCH a dramatic entrance—the "girls" and Dr. Molthrop (aka Dr. G.) would have loved it!

In addition to the popcorn, I also brought a TON of magazines. My godness-son, Justin, works in an advertising agency in New York City and when I was first diagnosed, he apparently told ALL of his clients that his godmother was diagnosed with breast cancer. So...for the past six months, I have received FREE subscriptions to Oprah, Elle Décor, Southern Homes and Gardens, Us, People, Self, Simple Life and Vanity Fair. The comment that was made by Sally in the front office was "Oh, so you think our magazines suck?"...to which I said..."UH-h-h, YEAH!!

Anyway....

I told the girls at the front desk that I "had run out of friends"...and I would be alone for my last treatment, so Kathy Lee (one of the "gals" at the front desk who really appreciates my humorous stories) gave me a ceramic bell and told me to "ring" it when I needed someone to help me—WHOA...WRONG MOVE!!! I don't have to tell you that I rang the bell when I weighed in at 129 (from 128 the week before)...rang it when I went in for my lab work...rang it when Dr. Molthrop came into the room to see me...and then rang it EVERY time someone said "Oh, so this is your last treatment??"

In addition to the goodies that I brought, I packed a picnic for me and my "CHEMO-SABE", Cheryl—who was also having her last treatment. I brought egg salad sandwiches (a good food item for chemo day) and ginger ale with two crystal champagne glasses that I had put in the freezer the night before.

Cheryl—who works at Ruth's Chris Steakhouse—brought two individual-sized banana cream pies topped with fresh banana slices—*to die for!!!*

The nurses placed a little TV table between us and I poured the "champagne" as we chowed down in a Benadryl and Decadron BLISS—while everyone else in the chemo room just smiled and shook their heads *(they're going to miss me when I am gone!)*

Four hours later, the chemo was finished!!! So, I heartily rang the bell and the girls (Kathy Lee and Sally) ran from the front desk as I yelled "I AM FINISHED!!! Then, I TOOK OFF MY WIG AND THREW IT UP IN THE AIR...just like Marlo Thomas in her "That Girl" series! Of course, everyone laughed and commented on "how good" I look without my wig and what a "great shaped head" I have. These are things I will long remember...

After I was awarded my "CONGRATULATIONS CERTIFICATE," I got up to leave, hugged all the nurses and patients and then went out toward the waiting room and hugged everyone there—and I was ringing my bell the whole time! *(they're gonna miss me when I am gone)*

Kathy Lee and Sally both gave me a hug and told me they loved me... and then, guess what they said?...

They said: "Give me back the damn bell!"

...but then they said: "We're going to miss you...Thursdays won't be the same without you!"

So, that ends my saga with the chemo. Now, I just have to deal with the wait for my hair to grow back (along with my eyebrows and eyelashes...all of which I have maybe 6 of each) AND two more surgeries and a tattoo...and maybe a face lift...or just a blepharoplasty...or hell, maybe just Botox. I haven't figured it out yet.

I do have my implant surgery scheduled for June 23rd (I know...here we go again)...but hopefully, that will be minor compared to past several procedures.

During my treatment I lost a total of 7 pounds...down to a size 4—without the butt—size 6 with the butt. However, I just want you to know I have regained my appetite...I used to realize at 9 pm that I hadn't eaten dinner, and now I realize that at 9 pm, I have been eating since 5:30pm!!

Well, I can't believe it; but, once again, I have written WAY too much—so, to all of you who have been telling me stories of your own Divine Interventions...I am happy that you have become aware of them and know that God has always been there—we all know the story of the "Footprints".

So, until the next time...keep praying for me and for the other 120,000 women who will be diagnosed with breast cancer this year. I appreciate—and will never be able to express to each and everyone of you—how much your support, care and encouragement has meant to me.

I love you!!

Carla

Dear Butterfly~
YAYYYYYYYYYY!
Love, Beth

Car~

Thanks a WHOLE lot for making me cry (with joy—for you and your incomparable sense of humor) just as I am ready to leave for work...now my eye makeup is running.

Congrats, congrats, congrats and God Bless.

You never had to convince me that He was always around. I have always believed that.

As to the numbers, I have heard (read, actually) that the number of new diagnoses this year is somewhere between 200,000 and 211,000. I hope you are right. But if not, may they all have an experience of love and support like you have had. You Go girl!

Love always ~ Maur

Carla,

I couldn't be happier for you. Your courage and fortitude during these trials is inspiring. I wish I could reach up and put my arms around you, but hopefully that will come soon. Wishing you speedy hair growth and an additional 10 lbs to fill out your butt.

Keep the faith and know that I think of you often.

Love, Pat D.

CJ - Do you think the (bleep)ers will miss you when you are gone? BRW

Carla~

This is WONDERFUL!! I just love it.

When are we doing the book? We need to do it SOON while everything is still fresh in your memory.

I love you! Trish

Our beautiful, funny, HEALTHY, Carla—

Your friends are so proud of you. I, for one, found myself being lifted up from what you were going through. You are one of the strongest women I know. I am very blessed to have you as a friend.

Now...about this butterfly party...I get to be an Orange one. I took a tour of a French butterfly farm—they eat bananas & exotic fruits (sipping adult beverages with tropical fruits count!) And they flit around from one beautiful flower to another...Lots of possibilities! Keep me posted!

Love you! Jennifer E.

Carla,

Thanks again for an awesome, inspiring and hilarious update. We are so happy for you and will continue to pray for you for a very, very long time. We hope to see you again soon, too!

Have a great weekend! We love you!

Jacqueline, Jeff, Ashton and Tristan

Carla,

Congratulations! Now you can look forward to surgery in June and you will emerge fully as that butterfly.

Speaking of butterflies, I was in New Smyrna last week and it is butterfly season there. They are everywhere!

Do you remember when we were there a few years ago and Marge rented that beach house? There were creamy white butterflies all over. Well, they're back! ...and so are you! Stay well.

Love, Barbara

Carla –

Congratulations on finishing your treatments! Your stories have been an inspiration, not to mention hilarious. You really ought to think about publishing your story. Talk about making lemonade...

I have been on the road constantly for months and months. Most recently, I left my home on May 6th and returned on May 28th. The whole family then boarded airplanes the next day for 10 days in Hawaii. Wow! It was fantastic.

I depleted the entire supply of red wine on the LA to Maui flight (imagine), so I arrived slightly dehydrated, but Hawaii was absolutely incredible. We had the best family time.

I don't know if LL is on your email list, but I know she would love to hear from you. You may know this, but her mother is in the final stages of ovarian cancer.

Also, I am going to see Pat D. in July. Coincidentally we arrive on July 22, which is Bruce's birthday. I am glad we will be there on that day—birthdays are hard, but at least it is not a "first". Pat is doing pretty well and is starting to emerge back into the world again. I know that your stories and your incredibly positive approach to your bout with cancer have really lifted her up. She always asks if I have seen your emails and reminds me that we need to keep you in our prayers, which we have and will continue to do.

Well, keep me posted on how you are doing and I hope to see you sometime.

Love, Jennie

Hi Jennie~

You sound VERY busy and I appreciate the time you took to send me the wonderful note. Hawaii sounds fabulous—I have an opportunity to go to Maui next February with a couple of friends of mine. One friend,

Priscilla, (the one I referred to in my last Metamorphosis email) has friends that have a condo there, so all living expenses would be provided for. I can't wait!

Regarding my emails to Lorraine—yes, she called me awhile back and we had a nice chat—it was then that I got your email address. I have been keeping Lorraine updated on my "progress". Many of those who have received my emails have encouraged me to publish...I wouldn't quite know where to start...but believe if it is something I should do...I will be guided toward that end and if it is meant to be, it will happen, I am sure.

I just got off the phone with a friend of a friend who was just diagnosed with breast cancer last Tuesday—41 years old with a 3 yr old. She is struggling with the diagnosis as she researches for information about what to do and who should do it. I just find myself wondering why SO MANY women get this? It's almost epidemic...

I would love to see Pat—she has been a great source of comfort during this challenging time...give her a GREAT BIG HUG from me when you see her.

Thank you for your continued prayers—the power of prayer is so significant in our lives.

Be well, my friend and God bless you always!

Love, Carla

Carla,

We were so thrilled with your last E-mail informing us of your final chemo session. Everything seems to be going well and in your favor. I can just see you throwing your wig up in the air, saying to the world: "I have overcome this obstacle. I am woman—hear me roar!"

We will continue to pray for you daily, offer our masses and communion, and light the candles every Saturday. So far our prayers have been answered. We have been feeling pretty good, little aches and pains here and there but nothing to worry about. These small inconveniences come with age and are to be expected. Take care and we'll talk with you soon.

Love, Mom and Dad

Dear Mom & Dad~

Thanks for all of your support and encouragement. I really meant it when I said I was going to quit after the second chemo. But, mom, you were the one that said to "buck up and just get through it."

I truly do believe in the power of prayer and I appreciate the many prayers you both have said for me.

Thanks also for the medals and the prayer cards and the candles and the masses, etc. etc. etc.

I love you both and hope to see you soon.
Carla

15. Getting Back to "Normal?"

There is a vitality, a life force, an energy, a quickening that is translated through you into action and because there is only one of you in all time, this expression is unique. And if you block it, it will never exist through any other medium and be lost. The world will not have it.'

—Martha Graham (1893-1991)

Date: 6/17/04
To: My Prayer Group
Subject: Metamorphosis - Part XV
Fuzzy Wuzzy was a bear...Fuzzy Wuzzy had no hair....Fuzzy Wuzzy wasn't fuzzy, was he?

Well, three weeks post-chemo and I am starting to get a little FUZZY! Actually, I can't tell if I am growing hair or have "prickly heat". I can see some little bumps (almost like goose bumps) all over my head. The fuzz is very light, so I can't tell if it is white or blonde. Kelly has scrutinized my scalp and seems to think that I have "blackheads" all over my head; so I am assuming the fuzz comes first and the dark hair later. But, since this process is one of learning, I guess I have to "wait and see" just as I have during much of this whole experience.

As I mentioned in my last email, I am having surgery to replace the expanders with implants next Wednesday, June 23rd at 4:30pm. I have decided (after speaking with several women with implants; some of whom are breast cancer survivors), that I am going to have the silicone implants. At this time, the FDA is only approving the silicone implants for women who have had mastectomies due to breast cancer, and as a result, I will be enrolled in a 5-year study to determine their safety, etc. Apparently, 30,000+ women are in the study so far, but the FDA wants more data.

After having read the 12-page informed consent forms, I was told that:

No, the manufacturer does not pay for any part of the study...or side effects or doctor's visits resulting from those side effects.

The manufacturer does not pay for any part of the surgery if the implants leak, explode or implode (Just kidding...I added the last "plode")

BUT...for $100.00, I can buy an EXTENDED WARRANTY on my implants to have them replaced if either of the first two occurrences happen.

How do you like that??? I am going to have a LIFETIME WARRANTY on my boobs!!!

I am also going to have my port removed....which is like having a huge tumor taken off my chest. (REALLY...it sticks out about ½ inch and it as round as a nickel!!) And, it will be nice to have the plastic surgeon suture the skin, so the scar won't be so noticeable. (As if THAT is my biggest worry! Ha!)

Anyway, he is also going to hike up my boobs a little, because he (and I) think that they are a little "low". (Not low as in tire pressure, but low as in horizontally on my chest).

Before I went to see Dr. Rotatori today, I stopped in to see my favorite ladies at Dr. Gorgeous' office...Sally and Kathy Lee. They screamed and ran out from behind their desks to hug me! I really miss those ladies! I went in to see the nurses also; but, I didn't get the same response (I never really bonded with the nurses....they made me SICK!!!! Get it???)

Yesterday, I dropped into my surgeon's office (Dr. Willard—you remember how much I love her!), and spoke to her nurse, Susie, who had breast cancer about 6 years ago...and she said: "You would not believe the number of women that are coming in and being diagnosed with Breast cancer."

I just don't get it....I can't tell if I am more aware of breast cancer because I had it (like being pregnant and noticing all of the pregnant women) or if this truly is becoming epidemic. Anyway, I pray each night that none of my friends or family ever have this experience and that I, myself, don't have to re-live it.

Let's wrap this up by talking about my most recent D.I.—I was driving past a church today and saw a sign in front that said: "Sorry, it is NOT all about YOU!!" I felt like God was speaking directly to me! But, then I thought...NO...he must be speaking to my Bunnie/JanJan!!!! So...heed that message, sistuh!!!

I don't really know if you want to continue hearing the details or if we should just end this communication...(and you can read the book when it comes out!!!) Keep the prayers coming and thanks for your continued concern and support.
Love you all!!!
Carla

After my chemo ended, and as I was starting to feel better, I assumed that "My Prayer Group" emails had run their course and my family and friends were tired of receiving my updates. I was working more and had less time (and less humorous stories) to convey, so I didn't send an email for about a month.

As I approached the date for what was to be my VERY LAST surgery, I thought I had things under control. But, once again my well-planned efforts were overthrown—probably just to make sure that I had learned my lesson: *In order to receive help, you must ask for it.* So yet again, my plea went out, asking for help.

> Date: 7/20/04
> To: My Prayer Group
> Subject: Metamorphosis –LAST Call for Help
> I just went to see the plastic surgeon and have scheduled my last surgery for Friday, August 27th at 11:00am at Florida Hospital Outpatient Center on Rollins.
> Originally, my plan was to have it the week before and based upon that plan, Kelly booked a flight to LA to visit a friend the last week of August (she had a ticket that had to be used before October). Needless to say, once again my desire to control things has been squashed. The August 20th surgery date is full and I have to delay one week to the 27th. Thus, my call for help.
> I will need someone to escort me to surgery (probably will have to be there at 9-9:15am) and someone to pick me up (probably about 7:30pm)...and an emergency phone number in that event.
> Also, it is necessary that someone stay with me that night (Friday) and Saturday night. I don't know whether I will need someone Sunday, but I would like to ask for that and if it's not necessary, we can cancel.
> You don't know how it pains me to ask this one more time...but I hope this is the last for a VERY long time. I am so grateful to you, my friends. I could not have done this without all of your support. I thank God for you each and every day.
> I love you all.
> Carla

Marge responded quickly to my request and offered to spend the entire weekend with me. In addition, Kay, Nadine and Diana offered their assistance. So, I decided to accept Marge's offer to take me to and from the hospital, and then have Kay and Nadine help me through the weekend. (We all remember that Diana—who is not a nurse—probably could not stand the site of blood, sutures or dressings. So, I just asked her to say some prayers for me.)

Date: Sunday, August 22, 2004 8:01 PM
To: My Prayer Group
Subject: Metamorphosis - Beauty is in the Eye of the Plastic Surgeon
Hello to All of my wonderful family and friends:
I just wanted to give you an update, since I have been remiss in doing that lately. I guess I didn't send anything following my last surgery (which was the port removal and implant replacement). I have healed nicely from that surgery, which was pretty much a non-event. I am so-o-o happy to have that damn port removed, that I actually forgot that the implants were part of the surgery!
Anyway, I have been doing well both at work and at home...still working out and maintaining my somewhat healthy lifestyle. I have had a few glasses of wine over the past few months; although I am giving it up these past 10 days, as I am preparing for what I hope is the last of my surgeries for many years to come.
I saw Dr. Gorgeous last week and he said that my blood work is back to normal and he will see me in 4 months. Of course, the girls at the front desk thought I looked FABULOUS!!!!
This Friday, I am having my final reconstruction on the breasts, which will replace what was removed during the mastectomies. Yes, in addition to that, I am having a mini face-lift and lower blepharoplasty (eyes), as I mentioned several months back. I figure, what the hell—may as well take advantage of having the plastic surgeon there—what's a few more hours?
I will be off work from Friday, August 27th until Monday, September 5th, so I will have a nice recovery/vacation. If you feel the urge to come visit me—I would love to have you come over...and will be happy to display the work of my artist.
Oh, by the way, I am in the process of writing a book to incorporate the emails that I have written over the past 10 months and would like to say that if you do not wish to have your name mentioned in it, please write back and let me know; otherwise the lack of your response will be taken as "permission granted".

Until the next time, please keep me in your prayers, particularly on Friday from 11:00am until about 6pm or so (through recovery) and I will "talk" to you soon after.
Love you all, Carla

Car,
I would love to have an autographed copy when all is said and done...my own expense of course.
Love,
Maur

Little did they know that their words of encouragement were the motivating force behind this book—and Maur, I put in your response...just to remind you that you owe me $16.99.

16. Weathering the Storm

Life is not a journey to the grave with the intention of arriving safely in a handsome and well-preserved body; rather, the objective should be to skid in broadside, thoroughly used up, totally worn out and loudly proclaiming: "WOW...WHAT A RIDE"
—Author Unknown

The year 2004 was an unforgettable one for me...as it was for all the residents of Florida.

Personally, I had survived bilateral mastectomies; surgery for a port placement, eight rounds of chemotherapy, port removal, implant surgery and nipple reconstruction, but now Mother Nature decided that she should also pack in a few punches...just to make life interesting!

One week prior to my final surgery—the second of what would be five hurricanes to hit Florida in one season—was making its way to Orlando. Bonnie had hit Pensacola and the upper west part of the peninsula; but Orlando was not impacted with that first hurricane. Hurricane Charley, though, was destined to make landfall in southwest Florida and then would cross directly over Orlando heading east. As it violently blew across the state, Charley's force was downgraded, but it hit my neighborhood at about 10:15 pm with 85 mph winds.

In the thirty years that I have lived in Florida, I have never experienced a storm that maintained hurricane force winds so far inland. Interestingly, the storm hit on the day that I originally wanted my surgery scheduled. I found out a week later that all elective surgeries had been cancelled that day. *(Another Divine Intervention?)*

Exactly one week after Charley hit, I went to the hospital to complete the reconstructive surgery on my breasts. In addition to the reconstructive surgery, I had decided that I "deserved" to have a little plastic surgery on my face, as well. Little did I know (nor did anyone for that matter) that only four days after my surgery, a *third hurricane*, Frances, would start moving slowly towards Florida—and she was the size of Texas!!!

Frances was moving along at about 10 mph with winds of 150mph; it looked certain that almost every square mile in the state was going to feel some impact of this storm.

As I was housebound, recuperating from surgery, I could only watch the TV in horror. *I was becoming panicked!*

There is a lot of preparation to be done when a hurricane of that magnitude is coming. Because Kelly was working in south Florida, and I was in no shape to lift furniture off the porch, I couldn't imagine how I was going to prepare for this storm.

I started calling friends at their workplace—none realizing that the storm was coming (they were working—not focused on the Storm reports as I had been—glued to the TV for days).

I called Steve, a friend in the neighborhood, to discuss my dilemma. He walked over to my house and quickly cleared my back porch of the patio furniture and carried it to my garage. *Check that off my list of things to do in preparation for the storm!*

The next day, my next door neighbor, Nick, placed plywood over my windows. *Another item checked off the list.* I could only watch and wait for the storm to hit.

Since I was scheduled to have my sutures out on the day that Frances was to make landfall, I placed a call to the plastic surgeon's office to see if I could come in a day early. They told me to come in at 8:30am on Thursday morning.

As I prepared to go to the doctor's office, I knew that I also had to stock up on the hurricane essentials: water, canned foods, peanut butter, bread, batteries, candles—and cash—none of which I had replaced after Charley.

Sitting on the treatment table in Dr. Rotatori's office, his nurse, Anne finished removing my sutures. Dr. Rotatori came in to examine me and commented on the quality of his own work. (I like that he is confident—and that the results were as good as he expected.) I mentioned that I had to go to the store to get stocked up on some "hurricane items".

He looked at me strangely and said: "You're going like that?" *(meaning: no wig, no makeup and with yellow, pink and purple bruises all over your face and neck?)*

I was quite matter of fact, as I answered: "What can I do? I can't put on a wig—it will rub the suture line along my ears, I can't wear make-up while the sutures are healing under my eyes, and I can't get rid of the bruises...yep, I am going just like this!"

I jumped off the table and gathered my belongings.

After leaving the office, needing to get some cash, I stopped at the bank and walked up to the ATM, where about ten people were standing in line. *People were staring at me.* My hair was about ½ inch long and I looked like Demi Moore when she buzz cut her hair in the movie, "GI Jane".

Feeling extremely self-conscious, I said to no one in particular: "I am playing a part in a re-make of the movie, GI Jane".

No one laughed—they just looked at me—probably thinking that I was a battered wife. *Oh well.*

Next, I went to the grocery store and then to the drug store...each time looking people in the eyes and smiling. I knew I looked horrible; but some of them even smiled back. I felt like I had on a Halloween mask, as if I was incognito. I guess I figured that no one I knew would EVER recognize me in *this* disguise.

Later that day, I sent an email to my family and friends, as I was coming down the home stretch to my recovery.

Date: September 2, 2004
To: My Prayer Group
Subject: Metamorphosis –The Final Surgery

A quick email to give you the lowdown on the closing "chapter" of this experience that we have all shared over the past many months.

Work has been going well...but, this week I am on "vacation" following—what I hope to be—my final surgery. (Nipple reconstruction with skin taken from my lower abdomen; a mini-face lift and my lower eyes done).

Having had the surgery last Friday, I am 6 days post-op. I must have had one hundred sutures from the top of my head to the top of my crotch!

I am feeling pretty good physically, although I look like Rocky—after about 8 rounds! The bruising wasn't as bad as I thought, but at day six, I am a nice color of golden yellow and salmon pink under my eyes, cheeks and neck and still pretty purple around my mouth.

My bikini cut on my abdomen has steri-strips and looks good. Up until today, I hadn't been able to check out the ta-ta's, because the dressings were *actually sewn onto the skin.*

I went this morning to have most of the sutures removed. They took the dressings off and un-sutured the "marshmallow-type" dressing that was holding the reconstructed nipple in place. Dr. Rotatori says everything looks great...good circulation and healing. He truly is an artist.

Now I am ready to "begin" my new life with vigor and health —and faith that this all had a purpose—and that I do with it what I should.

Thank you for all of the help you have given me these past 10 months...I am most grateful and will always keep you on my prayer list.
Love, Carla

Hurricane Frances was slowly...and I mean s-l-o-w-l-y... lumbering towards the east coast of Florida. Over a two-day period the meteorologists went back and forth as to where it would hit—Melbourne or Vero Beach. My daughter and I were trying to make the decision as to whether she should stay put in Okeechobee (45 miles west of Vero Beach) or come back to Orlando (45 miles west of Melbourne).

As the hurricane moved closer, we relied on the meteorologist's information that it would probably hit in the vicinity of Melbourne. So, I decided it would be better for Kelly to stay put and not deal with the traffic that would soon be crawling north on the Interstate. I didn't know until a day or so later that it was the wrong decision.

In the meantime, only 7 days post-op, I had to get ready for a hurricane predicted to create the strongest winds ever known to hit Florida. The fear of the unknown is always the worst and so I prepared the interior of my house as if the roof might be blown off—moving lamps to the floor, pictures off the walls, and pushing my sofa close to the windows. I didn't have much in my freezer (having lost everything when my power went out for 3 days with Hurricane Charley), but I wanted to use up everything that was in it. So, I baked the small bag of chicken and hard-boiled all the eggs in my refrigerator, and planned my menus for the next few days: baked chicken breasts, egg salad and/or peanut butter sandwiches and water. I filled my freezer with 7 bags of ice. Before I placed plastic over my computer and shut it down in preparation for the storm, I wrote an email to my out-of-state Prayer Group.

Date: 9/3/2004
To: My Prayer Group (outside Florida)
Subject: Preparing for Hurricane #2 (to hit Orlando)
Kelly is hunkered down in Okeechobee with her client and friend, Stephnye...and feels like they are as prepared as any of us. This hurricane has wobbled all over the place...we don't know where it will hit, but from the most recent information, it may now hit closer to Melbourne or a little north (which brings it closer to me). We just have to sit tight, as we have finished the preparations. My upstairs windows are boarded up thanks

to my neighbor, Nick. It's weird to sit up here at the computer at 3:15 in the afternoon and the rooms are dark.

The young guys who live across from me are diligently hauling debris to the dump from a huge pile which has been sitting in the cul-de-sac in front of my house since Charley hit. I guess all the neighbors figured it was a convenient place to pile tree trunks and branches, while waiting for the county to pick it up. It makes me feel 100% better that it is gone—because in 90mph winds, the debris would be like flying missiles.

Already this morning, I have been to Walgreen's, Publix, and Lowe's to get last minute items that I had forgotten.

The stores are crazy with tons of people making last minute preparations...many items are hard to find—C-Batteries are sold out everywhere—and people are standing in lines for 8-10 hours to get a few sheets of plywood for their windows. I got some caulk at Lowe's, so that Nick could caulk around my upstairs window, where the water came into the garage during Charley.

Believe it or not, I have gone to these stores WITHOUT my wig, NO make-up, stitches behind my ears and bruises all over my face. I have transitioned from the vain, self-absorbed woman; to an 'I don't really give a shit what anyone thinks of how I look!' young-looking gal...It's amazing to experience the freedom that this continuing metamorphosis seems to provide!

Also, I have told my plastic surgeon that once this healing is over, I will be listing my date of birth as 1-29-1961 and **know** that I can get away with it. Ha!!!

We have maybe another 24 hours before this thing hits, so my plan is to use Mom and Dad as our "check point". Once Kelly gets power back, she will call to "check in" with mom and dad and I will do the same to let them know how I am. I was afraid that within Florida, Kelly and I may not be able to communicate for days...so I am hoping that we can call out of state to find out what's going on with each other.

I may or may not communicate again before the storm— depending upon how things go here. I will shut down the computer tomorrow about noon, so I can unplug the power and cable and get some plastic on it. Other than that, I am hoping we can sit in our rockers some day and talk about the "big one" (or rather TWO) that hit us in 2004.

Continue the prayers...it looks like the winds have decreased a little...from 150 to 135! I know—but as Kelly says, I'll take 20 mph less anytime we can get it!!

Love to all. Carla

On Saturday at 11pm, Hurricane Frances, packing winds of 130mph (and gusts up to 165mph) rammed the vicinity of Vero Beach. Several days later, Kelly would tell everyone about the experience of hearing trees falling around the property where she was staying and sounds similar to a freight train moving by, as Frances took her good ole' time moving through the area. None of the horses were hurt and only one stall had some minor damage. However, when they came out the next morning, water as high as 3 feet was covering the fences in the lower pasture and, as they drove in to Vero Beach to use the phones, she said it looked like a war zone.

Twenty-four hours later, Frances arrived in Orlando and, although the winds were only 90 mph, it took the exact same path as Charley...the difference was that Charley went through in about 45 minutes and Frances took almost 2 hours to move through the area—creating much more damage.

I lucked out with Frances and didn't lose power or cable. Watching the hurricane coverage on TV and seeing the destruction that was caused by the wind and water, gives one a sense of awe at the lack of control that we have in our lives.

H-m-m-m...There's that message again.

However, after struggling through the preparations and then doing what needs to be done to clean up the damage, I realized that the neighborhood camaraderie and the celebration of our shared hope and strength are what life—and its challenges—are all about.

> Dear Carla the Magnificent,
>
> I just signed on after many days of being offline due to sick computer/sick family, and printed out all your emails to read leisurely with my feet up somewhere cozier than in front of my computer! Then...I realized I was running out of time to tell you how much you have been in our thoughts (post surgery, but especially with these mega-storms threatening you and yours); possibly I am too late and your computer is taking its siesta already but thought I'd try to do this communication thing anyway...
>
> YOU ARE MY HERO!!!!! Keep safe! After everything you have weathered this past 10 months, a little (okay, big) storm won't stop you, I know! However, we are praying that you have no further incidents requiring major labor—you deserve a break, for God's sake!!!
>
> We are thinking of you and sending sunny Tucson skies your way. Love you much, Beth

17. The Aftermath

God says: "I am your joy. Do not be afraid to be happy, for ever since I wept, joy is the standard of living that is really more suitable than the anxiety and grief of those who think they have no hope"—Karl Rahner

Date: November 11, 2004
To: My Prayer Group
Subject: Metamorphosis: The End and the Beginning

November 11, 2003... It's hard to believe that *one year ago today*, I was diagnosed with breast cancer.

My heartfelt thanks and sincere appreciation goes out to each and every one of you for your continuous love and support when I needed it most. Without you, I could never have lived each day of the past year without fear.

I am feeling FABULOUS! I am going to the gym 3 times a week and slowly gaining back my weight (not too much, though, I hope). Every morning, I thank God for my health, my family and my friends.

I am going back to the river for my WWWW (Wild Women's Weekend in the Woods), which is where this saga began only one year ago.

Again, my friends and I will celebrate our lives and those who are in them. We will make a toast to all of you who have been through this struggle with me and who have helped me to overcome the obstacles...and I will sit by the river and rejoice in the memories of its calm environment that assisted me in my guided meditations.

Today, I want to share with you, the beginning of my "book"—the Prologue. I have written about 60 pages (and it's quite difficult, let me tell you) —but with your prayers, may I be guided to write something that will inspire those who read it.
Love to all. Carla

When I wrote that email, I *was* feeling fabulous and the year really seemed to have gone by quickly. Yet, as I reflected on the prior year, I began to think about how time stood still on the day I was diagnosed and how it just couldn't go fast enough while I was moving through the process.

I remember counting each phase of the treatment as *one more step towards the goal of being healthy* once again. It was like watching the ball drop in Times Square on New Year 's Eve:

10- the surgery
9- the post-op visits
8- meeting with the oncologist
7- appointments with the plastic surgeon
6- the first round of chemotherapy treatment
5- losing my hair
4- the second round of treatment
3- reconstructive surgery
2- the last of the doctors' appointments (for at least 4 months)
1- the first visit to the beauty salon for a trim

And then—one day—it's over! *The celebration could now begin.*
However, instead of celebrating, I began to feel a subtle **feeling of loss**. After a full year of living through this process—the focus was no longer on my health. As a result, I had to re-focus on the day-to-day activities of living without the central theme of 'cancer' or 'treatment'—and without anyone else's daily concern about how I was doing.

I began to fear that I would 'forget' all that I had learned during this experience. As a cancer survivor, I wanted to remember.

So, I began to anticipate the arrival of my "anniversaries":

...the anniversary of my diagnosis
...the anniversary of each of my many surgeries
...the anniversary of my 1st and last chemo treatments

No one else seemed to share the memories...no one else remembered the anniversary dates...as far as everyone was concerned, it was over! The cancer was gone, the treatments were finished and life was back to normal.

Everyone who had helped me through this process—who had provided support and encouragement—all went back to their busy lives...*just as I was beginning to realize what I had been through.*

During my chemotherapy, I recall Nathan telling me that he had read about cancer patients becoming depressed after finishing their treatment. I remember brushing off that statement thinking: *"I have always been emotionally stable... that will never happen to me."*

But, shortly after the one year anniversary of my diagnosis, I started to feel "down in the dumps". It crept upon me slowly, almost unnoticeably. I recognized that something was not quite right when I was feeling less than excited during the Christmas holidays.

This feeling continued for about three months and along with it, I began to feel anxious and unable to sleep. It continued through my January vacation trip to Maui with Priscilla—I didn't understand how I could not feel excited about a vacation to Hawaii! I called out to God asking, *"What is happening to me?"* — and praying, *"I need Your help!"*

Upon returning from my Hawaiian vacation, Diana was ready to celebrate our birthdays together with our infamous pajama party—and I couldn't get excited about that!!! My birthday had always been cause for major celebration and partying—even after my surgeries the year before.

We did have a birthday pajama party; but my heart wasn't in it. I invited only my closest friends and went through the motions with short moments of enjoyment; but they were not long-lasting.

After my birthday, I was trying to decide if I should go to a psychiatrist for some help...thinking that maybe I needed some anti-depressants. Instead, I began to express what I was feeling and shared those emotions with several of my friends and family. Without any of them knowing what the others said, they all came to a similar conclusion and what they said to me made a lot of sense.

"You have been through a lot this past year...the diagnosis, the surgeries, the chemo...all of the physical changes. You approached each and every one of those hurdles with a strong and steady resolve."

They all speculated that going through this experience could be compared to any traumatic event in one's life. While living through it, you do what needs to be done to get through it; however, when it is over, your subconscious mind allows you to react, "to finally fall apart", so to speak...to feel the grief and to feel the depression.

Each time I heard a similar explanation, I realized the truth in it; however, I wasn't feeling any better.

One day at lunch, following an in-depth conversation with Sue and Jo, I explained to them my feelings of anxiety, fear and depression, which I could not shake. I told them about an experience that I had while on vacation in Hawaii with Priscilla.

On the third day that we were in Maui, we booked a boat trip and I would be going snorkeling for the first time in my life.

I was a little peeved that we had to get up at 5:20am to be at the dock by 7:00am—we were on vacation, for heaven's sake! Still half-asleep, we drove toward the marina in the early morning dusk. The weather did not look good. As the black clouds were rolling in, I did not have a good feeling about the day.

A couple of hours later, we were cruising out to the bay with the waves crashing against the side of the boat. The water was rough and several people with greenish faces were hanging over the boat rail...feeding their breakfast to the fish.

After some general instructions from the boat crew about how to use the mask and snorkel; those who were not losing their breakfast seemed to be excited about getting into their gear and going into the water. I did not share their excitement (nor was I vomiting, thank heavens).

Not being a strong swimmer I was in fact terrified to go out in the water; particularly on a morning that was dark and threatening to storm. Priscilla was about the tenth person to jump off the dive step. I watched her kick her swim fins and move away from the boat. When she was about 20 feet away, she shook her head and shouted: "It's really rough out here...you're not going to be able to do this!" Great...What a waste of time and money and—oh yeah, thanks for the vote of confidence, my friend!

But even with those discouraging words, Priscilla kept calling me to come into the water.

After stalling for about 15 minutes, a woman on the boat successfully encouraged me to go in.

"You will regret it if you don't at least try", she prodded.

I hesitated...then jumped in the water...and immediately panicked!

My breath came in short, halting intakes through the snorkel and I was afraid that I would inhale the water into my lungs. As I looked down about 30 feet to the floor of the bay, I realized that my fear of heights was also kicking in. As my panic became stronger, I just could not catch my breath. I quickly rolled over and took a breath with my head out of the water.

I looked around at all of the people who were seemingly having a wonderful time. Slowly, as I was treading water, feeling like an idiot, my rational mind was saying "You just spent $35.00 for this trip, and an extra $10.00 for the wetsuit. You will most likely not be making a trip to Hawaii anytime soon...you need to create an enjoyable experience!"

It took several minutes of talking to myself; but eventually I put my face in the water and forced myself to relax. My body began to float and I started to gently kick my feet. I looked down at the fish swimming beneath me and realized I wasn't going to fall down to the bottom of the bay.

The more I relaxed, the more peaceful I felt. At one point, I had a realization: *"this must be what it is like to die."* It wasn't a morbid thought, but more of a lesson, one in which I intuitively knew that fighting through a death experience could be painful and anxiety-producing—but, when you "let go and went with the flow", it would seem that the experience would be so much more peaceful. To me, this was another Divine Intervention.

As I was sharing this experience with Sue and Jo at lunch that day, I re-lived that morning in Maui along with the horrible feelings of panic and breathlessness.

On the drive home, I pondered the lunchtime discussion and tried to make some sense of the emotions that seemed to be smothering me.

Sitting in front of my computer that evening, I received an email from my friend, Olga. She had not known about my snorkeling experience in Hawaii—nor did she know about the feelings of anxiety or stress that I was having. But when she shared the following with me...it was an answer to my prayers...

DEEP WATERS by Os Hillman
Others went out on the sea in ships; they were merchants on the mighty waters. They saw the works of the Lord...
~ Psalm 107:23-24a

When you were a child, perhaps you may have gone to the ocean for a vacation. I recall wading out until the waves began crashing on my knees. As long as I could stand firm, the waves were of no concern to me.

However, as I moved farther and farther into the ocean, I had less control over my ability to stand. Sometimes the current was so strong it moved me down the beach, and I even lost my bearings at times. But I have never gone so far into the ocean that I was not able to control the situation.

Sometimes God takes us into such deep waters that we lose control of the situation, and we have no choice but to fully trust in His care for us.

This is doing business in great waters. It is in these great waters that we see the works of God.

The Scriptures tell us that the disciples testified of what they saw and heard. It was the power behind the gospel, not the words themselves, which changed the world. The power wasn't seen until circumstances got to the point that there were no alternatives but God. Sometimes God has to take us into the deep water in order to give us the privilege to see His works.

Sometimes God takes us into the deep waters of life for an extended time. Joseph was taken into deep waters of adversity for 17 years. Rejection by his brothers, enslavement to Pharaoh, and imprisonment were the deep waters for Joseph. During those deep waters, he experienced dreams, a special anointing of his gifts to administrate, and great wisdom beyond his years. The deep water was preparation for a task that was so great he never could have imagined it. He was to see God's works more clearly than anyone in his generation.

God had too much at stake for a 30-year-old to mess it up. So, God took Joseph through the deep waters of preparation to ensure that he would survive what he was about to face. Pride normally engulfs such young servants who have such access to power at such a young age.

If God chooses to take us into deep waters, it is for a reason. The greater the calling, the deeper the water. Trust in His knowledge that your deep waters are preparation to see the works of God in your life.

After reading this email, the tears began to flow—large, salty tears streaming from my eyes and dripping off my chin. I felt a release...a sudden understanding of what I had been through and I cried for the first time since the night I was diagnosed.

As I struggled to see through my blurry, tear-filled eyes, I wrote to my friends, thanking them for their insight and inspiration during the lunch; and sharing with them the Deep Water story.

Date: 1/31/2005
To: Sue and Jo
Subject: Deep Water

I want to thank you, Sue, for a very special afternoon. Your house looks absolutely beautiful...but, more than that, it FEELS beautiful...and peaceful...and full of the love that you and John so clearly put into it.

Today, for the first time in weeks, I am feeling more serenity than I have felt in weeks. Perhaps it was because you both helped me to acknowledge some feelings that I was unable to recognize. I am truly thankful to have both of you in my life—I feel as if you were sent to help me along in my journey and as I sit here, the tears are starting to flow—something I haven't done since the day I was diagnosed.

They are not tears of sadness, they are tears of relief and joy—knowing that no matter what happens in my life—I have friends who are willing to hear me and help me...and love me.

From the deep...deep part of me...I want to *Thank You Both So Much* for being there when I need you. I am truly blessed to have you in my life.

I love you both. Carla

P.S Another friend sent this to me this evening—I was touched by the meaning that it held for me...particularly after our conversation this afternoon.

> Carla...
>
> Many thanks for your email and inspiring attachment on "Deep Water"...beautifully said...I have made a hard copy of it to reflect upon again.
>
> I loved having you and Jo over...it felt good to host. Carla, I appreciate your open-hearted presence; your candor regarding your journey. Thanks for trusting & sharing that space of "deep waters". What you are expressing now seems so understandable to me—given the events of the last year/plus.
>
> It does occur to me, however, that these are "uncharted" waters for you (for most of us). But, then you must be getting a "nudge" from some source to explore it (the feelings).
>
> I look forward to our next gathering (wet suits and all—HA! for the deep waters)! Be easy with yourself...remember the sense/image of breathing easier and "letting go" while snorkeling.
> Love, Sue

A few weeks later, the depression and anxiety lifted. I am not sure how or why this happened. I do think that acknowledging the grief of the last year had something to do with the release of those emotions. And, I know that if they continued, I would have sought professional help because I did not want to continue feeling that way.

I have since been told that the sleeplessness may have been the result of having had six surgeries within an eight month period. In addition to having chemotherapy, the anesthesia obviously had some effect on me both physically and neurologically...and probably will for many months to come.

As they say, the worst part is over.

I will continue to live as a "survivor" as so many women before and after me, will do. A survivor keeps a positive attitude and believes that they have won the battle; but will continue to fight when necessary. Also, when help is needed and requested, it will be delivered. All of these things are possible through family, friends and prayer.

My support system continues and on occasion I am asked how I am doing. I know what that question means and so do others who have been touched by cancer.

Do I fear that my cancer will come back?

I know it is a possibility, but I do not focus on it. Instead, I try to live in the moment and treasure each day as a gift. I try to put things in perspective and not let the "little things" bother me. I try to remember that "everything is as it should be" and I will be perfectly fine...no matter what challenge Life decides to present to me.

One of the blessings that I received was seeing the love that is so abundant in my life.

I now see cancer in a new light and hope that I will always remember what I have learned from this experience.

As a result of having breast cancer, I am now part of a sisterhood that, otherwise, I would have never known. I share in a sisterhood that has experienced the tears that come with this diagnosis and its treatment; and I also experienced the laughter that refreshes the spirit, as it joyfully opened the way through those tears.

> Dear Carla: My thoughts and love are with you as you heal from your experience. I recently received this blessing from a friend and immediately thought of you.
> I love you, dear friend.
> Will call soon.
> Pat S.
>
> Written by Pat Bergen, CSJ
>   —Sister of St. Joseph, LaGrange, IL
> *Faithful God whose life flows through all the seasons*
> *Bless this woman.*
> *Breathe new life in her to renew*
> *and refresh her spirit.*

Warm her with cherished memories
and delight her in the wisdom she shares.
Be with her now as she opens her hands
in a spirit of letting go.
Let her heart hear the whispers
of new voices and new learnings.
May she know that she is loved
as she has loved.
Gift her with peace and
fill her with Your radiant joy. Amen.

What to Expect... Helpful Hints

Although I may have initially approached the diagnosis of breast cancer as a nurse...in the end, I believe I tackled it as a woman going through a new and difficult challenge. I don't pretend to believe that everything that I did during this experience was right. But, I can say that it *was right for me.*

If you or a loved one has been diagnosed with breast cancer, the following *may be helpful* to making your approach the right one for *you.*

It is important to take each step of this journey one at a time—dealing with what is happening in the present, rather than looking at what may or may not be in the future. This will keep you focused and less anxious.

Diagnosis. For me, the diagnosis was the most difficult phase of my experience with breast cancer. Being diagnosed with breast cancer is a shock, to say the least. When you add the fact that important decisions need to be made shortly after the diagnosis, a state of confusion follows. This confusion results from the lack of knowledge and control, and can lead to panic and/or depression if you don't 'get a grip" on what is happening to you. You tend to want others to make the decisions for you...but just know that *you must make them for yourself.* Given enough time and research, you **will** come to your decisions wisely and responsibly.

To get there, though, it is helpful to talk with others who have been through the experience and to become educated about the options for your treatment. The more you learn about your specific breast cancer "factors" (size of the tumor, grade, cell type, hormone receptor status, etc.) and its treatment, the more you will feel in control. Once you regain this sense of control, you will find the strength to make decisions, accept the diagnosis and begin to move forward with a treatment plan. From that day on ...it is one day at a time.

If you don't know anyone who has been through a breast cancer experience, ask your doctor if there are any previous patients who would be willing to talk with you. Keep in mind that your experience may be different than theirs; however, it will give you some idea of what to expect. Focus on the positive things that they experienced and those that will help you prepare for this journey. Shut out anything that you find to be negative (mind over matter), remembering that their negative experiences do not have to be yours.

A support group may also be an option for you to pursue at this time. The Cancer Center in your community will have information about local support groups. Most likely, the Center will also have a Breast Cancer Coordinator, a nurse who specializes in helping women find appropriate resources to deal with breast cancer treatment. (Read more about *Where To Find Support* on page 171.)

The internet is also an invaluable resource for educating yourself about breast cancer and its treatments. (See *Suggested Internet Resources* on page 174 for informational websites to assist you.)

Radiation. Due to the small size of my tumor and because I had bilateral mastectomies, I didn't need radiation. However, radiation therapy may be recommended to specifically rid the body of any microscopic cancer cells possibly remaining near the area where the cancer was originally found.

The usual course of therapy includes daily treatments five days a week for five to seven weeks, with each session lasting an hour or less. There is no nausea or hair loss from radiation therapy.

One of the more challenging issues with radiation therapy is arranging it to fit into your work schedule, because it is administered daily. You will be able to drive yourself back and forth, though, since the therapy has no debilitating side effects. Generally, the drive to and from the Center is longer than the actual treatment.

After a few weeks of radiation, the most common side effects may include reddening, dryness and itching of the skin. Few patients develop significant irritation which usually heals completely within a few weeks of completing radiation treatments.

Surgery. If you are told that you need a biopsy for a breast lump, my recommendation would be to find a surgeon who is well-known in your community for treating breast cancer patients. If the biopsy comes back positive for breast cancer and the tumor margins are not clear (meaning that there are cancer cells along the *edge*s of the tissue), the experienced surgeon will have left "markings" on your remaining breast tissue in order to know where the lump was situated prior to removal. This way, if you must go back in for a lumpectomy or quadrantectomy, your surgeon will be able to locate the area where the cancer cells extended beyond the edges of the biopsy site. The amount of breast tissue removed depends on the size and location of the tumor. If 20 percent to 25 percent of the breast is removed, the procedure is called a quadrantectomy.

If you have the choice of either a lumpectomy, quadrantectomy or single or bilateral mastectomy, be sure to make your decision based on your research along with your "gut instincts", being certain that you are comfortable with that decision.

Chemotherapy. Chemotherapy affects the whole body because it goes through the bloodstream to kill rapidly dividing cancer cells that may have spread to other parts of the body. Chemotherapy treatment protocols may differ from patient to patient, depending upon the breast cancer "factors". Your doctor will determine the best treatment protocol for you; but it is important for you to understand the chemotherapeutic agent that will be given. Different types of chemotherapy produce different side effects—but each can be treated effectively with medications. Side effects of chemotherapy come about because cancer cells aren't the only rapidly dividing cells in your body. The cells in your blood, mouth, intestinal tract, nose, nails, vagina, and hair are also undergoing constant, rapid division. This means that the chemotherapy will affect them, too.

Hair loss, fatigue and nausea are some of the more common (and annoying) side effects resulting from the administration of chemotherapy.

Side Effects. *Hair loss* can be one of the most devastating side effects of chemotherapy; however, there are things you can do to make it less upsetting. When you are diagnosed with breast cancer and told that you will be having chemo, have your hair cut shorter. If you have long hair, you may want to go to shoulder length or even shorter. This way you will be "sporting a new do" prior to your chemo treatments. Once you have the new hairdo, go to a wig store to be fitted with a wig that looks the same as or similar to your new hairdo. Rachel Welch has a line of beautiful synthetic wigs that run about $135 each. Synthetic wigs are easier to care for (and less expensive) than wigs made with real hair. Check your health insurance policy to see if your insurance company will pay for the wig. If not, ask the wig store for a "breast cancer discount". If you can't afford a wig, the American Cancer Society has resources and may be able to get one for you. Some women prefer to wear scarves or hats and do not bother with a wig. Decide what your preference is prior to having the chemo. And, if you choose to get a wig, do two things: take it to a hairdresser who has experience in trimming wigs to make it look more like your own; and *fit the wig to your head* by stitching the web inside the wig. Nothing looks worse than a wig *that looks like a wig*!!!

After starting chemo, you will begin to lose your hair within approximately three weeks. When you start noticing a lot of hair in your shower drain or on your pillow...go to your hair dresser and ask them to give you a buzz cut, leaving about ¼" of growth (to prevent infection from a closer cut). This will relieve your anxiety about watching it fall out in clumps...and it will be time to start wearing your wig.

You may or may not lose your eyelashes and eyebrows...it was only after my 7th treatment that mine started to fall out. I went to the MAC counter in my favorite department store and had the cute little salesperson show me how to put on false eyelashes and draw on eyebrows...but the eyelashes became a hassle, so I only wore them about 3 times. I got really good at drawing on my eyebrows though. To this day, people tell me that they didn't realize they had fallen out!

Also, when your hair starts growing back (about three months after treatment ends)...it may come in with a different texture than you originally had. My straight hair came back in very tight curls while my friend's—who had curly hair prior to chemo—grew back stick straight! For me, the curls gradually softened and I ended up with hair that has nicer body than once did (my hairdresser loves it!).

Nausea results directly from the chemo which kills cells lining the gastrointestinal tract. Your doctor will prescribe anti-nausea medications, such as Zofran, Kytril or Emend; however, in addition to those, you may want to stock up on Zantac, Tagamet, Pepcid, Rolaids and Tums...these are over the counter medications that can be taken everyday (several times a day) to treat the "waves of nausea" that continue after you are finished taking the 3 day post-chemo treatment of Zofran, Kytril or Emend.

Fatigue is almost always a side effect of breast cancer treatment, resulting from a lower red blood cell count. Red blood cells carry oxygen through your system, so less red blood cells means you are getting less oxygen to your tissues and therefore you feel tired. When you feel tired, it's important to lie down and rest. However, when you feel better, try focusing your energy on quality things and some good physical activity. Get a family member or a friend to clean the house, go to the grocery store, or prepare meals that could be frozen and heated later. If others help you with some of the routine household chores, then you can focus on doing some things that are enjoyable and fun!

What You Can Do...

- *Learn about your cancer.* Read about your cancer to help you understand the disease process and its symptoms. Once you understand the disease, you can develop techniques to help you cope with (and sometimes avoid) the side effects and learn to adjust to the treatments. Write down questions about things that you don't understand and those that concern you.

- *Talk to your doctor.* Work together with your doctor on understanding and treating the disease. Discuss with him/her your questions and your concerns. Let your doctor know what you expect from him/her and your determination to be well. Be an advocate for yourself.

- *Seek support from your family and friends.* Some family members may experience feelings of helplessness, guilt, fear or anger. You and your doctor can help reduce these feelings by acknowledging that they are common in families of persons with cancer, and by encouraging your family's participation in your treatment. Of course, this involvement should be respectful of your privacy and independence.

- *Take control.* People with cancer are often passive and dependent in their healthcare. For example, they may decrease their physical or social activities, or depend on others to make treatment decisions. Increased activity and involvement will help you feel that you are in charge of your illness and your life. If you are unsure of how much activity you can handle, consult your doctor.

- *Consult a mental-health professional, if needed.* Consider counseling if: you are experiencing a co-existing psychiatric problem that requires treatment (e.g. severe depression); you need stress management; your psychosocial functioning is seriously impaired (e.g. you cannot participate in social activities); or marital or family problems are affecting your adjustment to the illness. Do not hesitate to seek long- or short-term counseling if you feel it will benefit you.

How to Cope

There are many things that you can do to be sure that you have the physical and emotional strength to cope with your disease and its treatment. One recommendation is to get on a regular schedule. Having a regular routine is critical to relieving stress in everyone's daily life. Rest is also very important. You need to make sure that you get a full night's sleep every night. If possible, a 30-45 minute daytime nap can also give you an energy boost. You should let your doctor know if you are having any difficulties sleeping.

If you have a stressful job, you may need to make some changes to lessen your workload. The same holds true for a hectic home life. Other family members may need to take over some of the responsibilities. Temper your physical activities to those that you can tolerate without placing undo stress on your body or increasing your symptoms.

Those who experience few symptoms with treatment may want to incorporate mild "exercise' into their daily or weekly routine. This can help to increase your stamina and reduce associated feelings of fatigue or tiredness. The long-term benefits of exercise can include reversal of muscle weakness and wasting, and prevention of calcium and protein loss from your bones. However, it is important to check with your doctor before starting any kind of fitness program.

Stress, Depression & Anger

Having breast cancer can be very stressful and sometimes downright depressing. Some of your coworkers or friends may not understand your treatment regime and therefore may change their attitudes toward you. You may feel somewhat isolated because your friends and family don't realize what you are going through or how you feel. As for anger, of course you're mad!!! It's not fair that you got this disease and NO...you do not deserve it.

Perhaps the most important thing you can do to cope with breast cancer treatment is to have a positive attitude. Replacing negative thoughts with positive ones is easier said than done, but it will make a difference in how you cope with your treatment. Increasing your activity level and making yourself smile more often are ways to start feeling better about yourself.

Many people also have looked beyond traditional medical care to find relief for their treatment side effects. For the symptoms of stress and depression in particular, many cancer patients have used stress management and relaxation techniques, including the following:

- *Meditation.* There are many different meditation methods, but they all work to quiet the mind and make you feel more peaceful and relaxed.

- *Yoga.* This is a slow stretching exercise that tones the body and relaxes the mind.

- *T'ai Chi.* One of the Asian martial arts that is different from judo or karate. The movements are slow and energizing, and, like yoga, it relaxes you as well.

- *Relaxation tapes.* There are wide varieties to choose from. Some are musical; others have guided medication. Choose a tape that works for you.

- *Journal writing.* Recording your thoughts in a journal often helps, especially when you do not feel comfortable discussing certain issues with friends or family. In addition to writing about your thoughts and feelings, you can keep track of your progress and list your goals so that you can see that you're taking control.

Where To Find Support...

Now that you have been diagnosed with breast cancer and are learning more about the disease, you may be thinking about how you should share this information with family members and friends you trust. These are the people who know you best and care about you the most, but it may be hard for you to talk about having cancer, especially at first.

Having to tell people about your condition and wondering whether they will care enough to try and understand can be scary. But it's a very important and rewarding step when your family and friends learn about something as important as this, and you realize you have people who are willing to help you.

For one thing, having someone to talk to who understands what you are going through will be a big help to you emotionally. But there are also practical reasons for telling someone you trust and can rely on about your condition. Family and friends can help you with daily concerns such as household chores, doctor's visits, eating healthy foods, and making sure you have the medications you need on hand.

In particular, you may need help taking care of your children if your symptoms become overwhelming.

- Think about your childcare needs both everyday and emergency. Then decide if you can ask some nearby friends or family members if your children can stay with them if you suddenly become ill.
- Make sure that the emergency contact information at the offices of your children's schools is up-to-date.
- Make sure that you explain your illness to your children in terms that they can understand, depending on how old they are. You should think about the same for anyone else, such as an elderly parent, whom you are taking care of now.
- Also, you may want to make arrangements for someone to take care of pets or other possessions, such as plants or valuables that are important to you, if you are unable to do so for a length of time.

If you feel you will need a lot of help, seek it out. Look into resources you may have, such as local agencies, support groups, or the members of your church, temple, or synagogue. Don't be shy about telling your pastor, priest, or rabbi about your illness. He or she can pray with you, give you advice, and help you come up with good plans for the future. Telling someone you have cancer may seem tough, but picking the right people to tell and giving them good information may help you. However, you also must consider how your illness will affect your ability to support yourself.

Support groups

Support groups have long been known to help their members cope with a health issue that has personally affected their lives. Many people have found that joining a support group provides them with the knowledge and information that they need to feel "in control" of their situation.

Additionally, support group members share their stories and experiences, making those who join a group feel that they are not alone. Support groups are appropriate forums to vent anger and guilt and fear about a situation that has changed their lives. The clinical and social benefits of support group attendance are well known—the numbers of patients and families who attend educational and supportive meetings are a testimony to the impact on the lives of those with cancer.

Many of us have witnessed firsthand how members benefit from the group atmosphere and enjoy an improved quality of life in the presence of cancer. Members' anxieties have been allayed, patients have become more compliant with their treatment regimes and not infrequently, medical outcomes have been positively impacted.

Mutual support groups have been found to be extremely effective in the management of a variety of chronic illnesses and are increasingly being recognized as viable, effective tools to supplement and extend the present physical health and mental health system.

Former Surgeon General C. Everett Koop stated: "I think that eventually self-help will be the 'other' health system in this country and it will accept the burden of disease awareness & prevention, and of heath promotion in the United States."

To find a support group near you, you may call your local Breast Cancer Treatment Center or the American Cancer Society. If you give them your zip code, they will give you the location of the nearest support group. You can reach them at 800-ACS-2345.

Memories of Your Experience...

Believe it or not... there are things about this experience that you will not want to forget. I suggest that you do one or more of the following:

1. Keep a "Grateful Journal"- writing in the names and thanking those who helped and supported you throughout your treatment.

2. Make a scrapbook – of all the notes and cards you receive, as well as other items (such as hospital name bands) that you want to save as memorabilia.

3. Take pictures! - before, during and after your treatment. You will look back on them one day, not believing what you actually went through.

4. Keep a journal of all the experiences that you have- document your emotions, both positive and negative.

5. Save all of your emails and those from your friends and family.

6. Take note of all of the people you meet and the things that happen (Divine Interventions) while you walk through this journey...and know that you are never alone!

Suggested Internet Resources

http://www.healthjourneys.com – Meditation, guided imagery and affirmations. Audio resources for the mind, body and spirit.

http://www.livingwithit.org/breast - Sponsored by Aventis Pharmaceuticals, the goal of the "Living with it" program is to provide information to women with breast cancer. If you enroll in the "Living with it" program, they will send materials via the U.S. mail to include:
- Information that helps give perspective on living with breast cancer
- A "Things to Keep" binder filled with resources and information about breast cancer
- Two additional mailings of program materials (sent 4 to 6 weeks apart)
- Additional information on lifestyle, diet & exercise, medical options, clinical trials, and insurance issues.

http://www.curetoday.com/freesubscriptions/index.html - This site offers free subscriptions to the Cure Magazine. Review the October 2003 edition on-line for information about breast cancer.

http://www.lookgoodfeelbetter.org – Provides information for women going through chemotherapy. Tips on skin care, makeup and wigs.

http://www.susanlovemd.com – Sponsored by the Dr. Susan Love Research Foundation, a nonprofit organization dedicated to ending breast cancer in the next ten years. This site has tons of information on breast cancer research and has answers to many of the questions that you will have about breast cancer and its treatment.

http://www.nlm.nih.gov/medlineplus/breastcancer.html- Sponsored by the National Institutes of Health, Medline Plus provides the latest news on breast cancer and its treatments.

http://www.cancer.org – Sponsored by the American Cancer Society, go to the "Choose a Cancer Topic" for specific information about breast cancer.

http://www.breastcancer.org – A nonprofit organization for breast cancer education, this site offers open chat rooms, discussion boards and information about community support groups.

http://www.komen.org - The nonprofit Susan G. Komen Breast Cancer Foundations sponsors "On the Way to the Cure" —educational outreach tours for the public. To learn more about them or if you have questions about breast cancer visit this website or call its national toll-free Breast Care Helpline at 1-800-462-9273.

http://www.mskcc.org/mskcc/html/44.cfm - Sponsored by the Memorial Sloan-Kettering Cancer Center, this site offers information on all types of cancer, including the latest breast cancer information.

http://www.mdanderson.org/diseases/BreastCancer - Sponsored by MD Anderson Cancer Center, this site provides up-to-date research information on breast cancer and its treatments.

http://www.radiologyinfo.org/content/therapy/thera-breast.htm - This public information Web site was developed and funded by the American College of Radiology and the Radiological Society of North America to inform and educate about radiology procedures, including radiation therapy for breast cancer.

References:

[1]Healing Touch International: www.healingtouch.net
Healing Touch is a biofield therapy that is an energy based approach to health and healing. It uses touch to influence the human energy system, specifically the energy field that surrounds the body, and the energy centers that control the energy flow from the energy field to the physical body. These non-invasive techniques that utilize the hands to clear, energize, and balance the human and environmental energy fields thus affecting physical, emotional, mental, and spiritual health and healing. It is based on a heart-centered caring relationship in which the practitioner and client come together energetically to facilitate the client's health and healing. The goal in Healing Touch is to restore harmony and balance in the energy system placing the client in a position to self heal.

Healing Touch complements conventional health care and is used in collaboration with other approaches to health and healing.

[2]Image Paths, Inc. of Ohio has been producing the Health Journeys (Website www.healthjourneys.com) audio series since 1991, making its award winning audiotapes and CD's available for retail distribution, and to pharmaceutical companies, hospitals, insurance carriers, governmental health facilities and direct mail customers. Health Journeys have been found effective in studies at UC Davis Medical Center, Memorial Sloan-Kettering, The Cleveland Clinic, and other Medical facilities.

[3]A PCA pump is a way to self-administer pain medication following surgery. The medication is suspended in an IV pump and delivered in small, but consistent doses once the patient presses the button. The doctor orders the amount of medication and the nurse adjusts the pump rate to limit the total amount of medication that a patient can self-administer. If I had pressed the button too often after having reached the medication dose ordered, the pump would not administer any more medication. At that point, if the patient continued to have pain, they would need to notify the nurse for additional pain medication or a different type of medication.

[4]Harold S. Kushner; author of the book: "When Bad Things Happen to Good People".

[5]*The Message from Water* was first published in June 1999 in Japan and sold more than 60,000 copies in less than a year. Although there has not been any commercial advertisement outside of Japan, the demand overseas was enormous, and Hado Publishing BV was set up in The Netherlands to meet the demand. More pictures may be viewed at www.hado.net. The book may be ordered via the following website: www.global-light-network.com or from the publisher at: Hado Publishing BV, Prinsenstraat 55, 2316 HK Leiden The Netherlands, tel&fax: +31-71-521-0897, E-mail: book@hado.net

[6]SeaCure® helps the digestive tract recover from injury and infection as well as cope with stress more effectively. If you are taking antibiotics or chemotherapy drugs, then your digestive system is under enormous stress. SeaCure® helps strengthen the digestive system so it can cope with the stress it is under.
http://www.naturedoc.com/information/seacure.htm

www.ingramcontent.com/pod-product-compliance
Lightning Source LLC
Chambersburg PA
CBHW020420290526
45785CB00002B/652